OVERCOMING HIGH BLOOD PRESSURE

OVERCOMING HIGH BLOOD PRESSURE

THE COMPLETE COMPLEMENTARY HEALTH PROGRAM

DR SARAH BREWER

WATKINS PUBLISHING
LONDON

Natural Health: Overcoming High Blood Pressure

For my wonderful husband, Richard

This edition first published in the USA and Canada in 2013 by
Watkins Publishing Limited
PO Box 883, Oxford, OX1 9PL
UK

A member of Osprey Group

Osprey Publishing
PO Box 3985, New York, NY 10185-3985
Tel: (001) 212 753 4402
Email: info@ospreypublishing.com

Commissioning Editor: Grace Cheetham
Managing Editor: Sarah Epton
Editors: Kesta Desmond and Rebecca Sheppard
Managing Designer: Clare Thorpe
Commissioned artwork: Mark Watkinson

ISBN: 978-1-78028-711-9

10 9 8 7 6 5 4 3 2 1

Typeset in Ehrhardt and Calluna
Printed in China

Publisher's note:
The information in this book is not intended as a substitute for professional medical advice and treatment. If you are
pregnant or are suffering from any medical conditions or health problems, it is recommended that you consult a medical
professional before following any of the advice or practices suggested in this book. Watkins Publishing Limited, or
any other persons who have been involved in working on this publication, cannot accept responsibility for any injuries
or damage incurred as a result of following the information, exercises, therapeutic techniques or recipes contained in
this book. The availability of some over-the-counter herbal remedies may be affected by the 2004 EU Directive on
Traditional Herbal Medicines. Consult a pharmacist or qualified herbal practitioner for advice on this subject.

Notes on the recipes:
Unless otherwise stated: use large eggs and medium fruit and vegetables. Use fresh ingredients, including herbs and
chilies. Do not mix metric and imperial measurements. 1 tsp. = 5ml, 1 tbsp. = 15ml, 1 cup = 240ml

Watkins Publishing is supporting the Woodland Trust, the UK's leading woodland conservation charity, by funding
tree-planting initiatives and woodland maintenance.

www.watkinspublishing.co.uk

Author's acknowledgments:
I would like to thank my husband, Richard, who willingly provided invaluable back up and support during those long
hours of research and writing. I would also like to thank everyone who has helped in bringing this book to fruition,
including Grace Cheetham at Duncan Baird, Judy Barratt and Kesta Desmond – who ensured consistency throughout
– and, of course, my inimitable agent, Mandy Little.

CONTENTS

INTRODUCTION

High blood pressure is an insidious condition that creeps up on you with little warning. As a result, one in three American adults has hypertension, yet at least half are unaware they are affected. This means an estimated one in six adults is walking around with an undiagnosed condition that can have serious effects on their long-term health—one in six of all your friends and relatives could be affected. Although you might have picked up this book for your own benefit, please encourage everyone you know to have their blood pressure checked if they haven't done so in the past year—they might be surprised at the result.

When hypertension is diagnosed, treatment is important as high blood pressure hastens the hardening and furring up of your arteries, which increases blood pressure even more. It's a vicious circle that can, if uncontrolled, eventually lead to coronary heart disease, a stroke, impaired vision, kidney problems, and poor circulation throughout your body—all from a condition that doesn't, in itself, make you feel unwell. Because high blood pressure is so potentially dangerous, it's important it's monitored regularly and that you aim to keep your blood pressure below 130/80 mmHg.

Although drugs are often needed to lower blood pressure, dietary and lifestyle changes can help bring down blood pressure significantly. In many cases, these changes mean you won't have to take anti-hypertensive medication at all. And, if you're already taking drug treatment, dietary and lifestyle changes can lower your blood pressure enough for your doctor to start weaning you off the medicine you're taking.

This book provides all the information you need to help keep your blood pressure within safe limits. It gives you information about the important dietary and lifestyle changes you can make, why regular exercise is so important, the benefits of relaxation, and the natural health approaches that work. These approaches might be new to you. Rest assured that the information given is based on compelling clinical research. I have included only those complementary therapies, food supplements, and dietary approaches that have the best possible chance of controlling your blood pressure naturally and safely.

Everyone is different and no diet and lifestyle plan will suit all individuals. For that reason, I've drawn up three different approaches: gentle, moderate, and full-strength programs, one of which is likely to suit you. To help you work out which plan is right for you, answer the detailed questionnaire on pages 109–111. This will point you in the right direction.

For those who want to take things slowly, the gentle program introduces you to healthy eating principles, such as cutting back on refined carbohydrates, cooking without salt, lowering your consumption of red meat, and eating more fruit, vegetables, and fish. Low doses of food supplements are also suggested. The gentle plan gets you stretching and walking and introduces you to complementary health approaches, such as aromatherapy, homeopathy, meditation, and yoga. The gentle program has the potential to lower your blood pressure by at least 4/2 to 7/4 mmHg within 30 days.

For those who want more of a challenge, or who are already following a relatively healthy diet and lifestyle, the moderate program introduces you to a wider variety of wholegrains, bean sprouts, and fruit and vegetable juices, and includes more of the superfoods shown to have beneficial effects on blood pressure. I suggest more therapeutic doses of supplements, and a more intensive exercise program. In addition, I introduce you to complementary approaches, such as qigong, herbal medicine, reflexology, and more advanced relaxation techniques. The moderate program has the potential to lower blood pressure by at least 7/4 to 11/5 mmHg within 30 days.

For those who already eat healthily and are very physically active, I recommend the full-strength program. This includes a diet based on seven superfoods identified as having the most significant beneficial effects on circulatory health. Supplement doses are suggested at the higher end of the therapeutic range. I also introduce you to naturopathy, acupuncture, and relaxation techniques, such as transcendental meditation. The full-strength program has the potential to lower your blood pressure by at least 15/8 mmHg over the course of just one month.

This book takes a holistic approach and is designed to complement the treatments your doctor prescribes. It is intended to offer general information, not to replace individual advice from your own doctor or other healthcare professionals who know your individual needs. Never stop taking your anti-hypertensive medication without your doctor's permission. Once your blood pressure starts coming down as a result of diet and lifestyle changes, your doctor should be happy to consider reducing your prescribed medication under careful medical supervision.

The information in this book is not intended for women who have high blood pressure during pregnancy. Never take food supplements or herbal remedies during pregnancy unless advised to by a doctor, pharmacist, or qualified medical herbalist.

To accompany this book I have created the following website: www.naturalhealthguru.co.uk. It features updated information, new recipes, and the most recent research findings. Please visit the site regularly to tell me how you are doing with the programs, and, most importantly, to share your successes.

LOOK OUT FOR THESE SYMBOLS

Throughout this book I have included boxes that highlight useful, interesting, or important pieces of information. Each box bears a symbol (see below). The arrow symbol indicates that a box contains practical instructions. The plus sign means the box contains additional information about the subject being discussed, or about high blood pressure in general. The exclamation mark indicates a warning or a caution.

PART ONE

UNDERSTANDING HIGH BLOOD PRESSURE

High blood pressure—or hypertension—can often be difficult to perceive as a serious medical condition. You might have been diagnosed with it, yet feel healthy. To fully understand high blood pressure, I think it helps to have some basic knowledge of the workings of the heart and blood vessels. In a healthy body blood pressure rises and falls throughout the day—a process that is facilitated by nerve signals, hormones, and other chemicals. The development of hypertension means that instead of fluctuating normally, your blood pressure stays high all the time. I explain the two different types of hypertension and the risk factors associated with each. If you have hypertension, it's important to know about the long-term complications, such as coronary heart disease, so you can take action to prevent them and be aware of their early signs and symptoms. The action you should take when you receive a diagnosis of hypertension depends on how high your blood pressure is—there are different categories that range from stage 1 (mild) to stage 3 (severe). Your doctor will decide whether you can manage your blood pressure through diet and lifestyle changes, or whether you need pills.I describe the range of medication you might be offered and explain how each treatment works.

WHAT IS BLOOD PRESSURE?

To function, all the tissues and organs in your body need a constant supply of oxygen and nutrients. These are supplied by your blood, which is pumped by your heart through a complex network of arteries and veins. The pressure at which your blood travels through your arteries is very important. If it is too high, it can damage or rupture a blood vessel, or result in bleeding in the brain. In the long term it can damage your organs. If blood pressure is too low, not enough blood—and therefore not enough oxygen and nutrients—reaches your body tissues and organs. If you've ever experienced low blood pressure as a result of standing up suddenly, you'll know that the main symptom is feeling faint. This is because the blood pressure in your arteries is temporarily too low to carry sufficient oxygen to your brain.

THE RISE AND FALL OF BLOOD PRESSURE

Compare the flow of blood through your blood vessels to the flow of water through a hose, for example. The water pressure inside a hose can vary from high to low, depending on factors such as how fully you turn on the faucet or whether you constrict the hose by squeezing it or inserting a blockage into it. The blood pressure inside your arteries rises and falls in a similar way. For example, if your heart beats faster and pumps out more blood, your blood pressure rises. If your blood vessels constrict or dilate, your blood pressure rises or falls respectively.

Your blood pressure fluctuates naturally throughout a 24-hour period. It is lowest when you are asleep (usually around 3 a.m.), and highest in the morning from the time before you wake to approximately 11 a.m. During your waking hours, your blood pressure goes up and down in response to a variety of factors. Anything that changes your cardiac output (the amount of blood pumped through your heart over a set period of time) will have an impact on your blood pressure. For example, exercise increases your cardiac output and causes your blood pressure to rise; so do anxiety, excitement, high environmental temperatures, eating, and cigarette smoking. Obesity increases your cardiac output and,

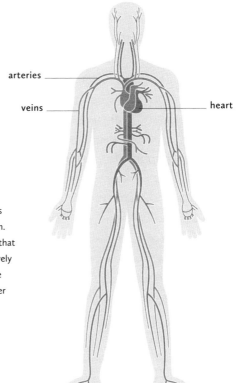

arteries

veins

heart

THE CARDIOVASCULAR SYSTEM
The heart, arteries, veins, and capillaries
(the tiny blood vessels that connect arteries
to veins) make up the cardiovascular system.
The arteries are strong and flexible vessels that
carry blood away from the heart at a relatively
high pressure. Veins carry blood back to the
heart at a lower pressure—they have thinner
walls and larger diameters than arteries.

therefore, your blood pressure. Even drinking a cup of coffee can cause a temporary spike in blood pressure.

These rises in blood pressure are completely normal—they are part of the daily rhythm of your cardiovascular system. Even if you run upstairs, go for a jog, or encounter some highly stressful moments in your day, your body quickly restores your blood pressure to normal afterward. It's only when your cardiovascular system stops working properly (with age, for example) that high blood pressure becomes a problem—instead of rising and falling in a regular, predictable pattern it stays high all the time, even when you're sitting still. This permanent state of high blood pressure can damage your body and is known as hypertension (see pages 17–22).

UNDERSTANDING BLOOD PRESSURE READINGS
Between each heartbeat your heart rests briefly. During this rest the upper chambers of your heart fill with blood, and your blood pressure is

at its lowest point—this is known as diastole. Almost immediately afterward, your heart contracts to push blood out into your arteries. As a result, your blood pressure rises—this is known as systole.

When you have your blood pressure taken, the reading yields two numbers that are written one over the other: the first is your systolic blood pressure and the second is your diastolic blood pressure. Blood pressure is measured in millimeters of mercury, which is abbreviated to mmHg (Hg is the chemical symbol for mercury). So if you have a blood pressure reading of 120/80 mmHg, this means your systolic pressure is 120 and your diastolic pressure is 80. When spoken, this is usually expressed as "120 over 80." This reading is typical for a healthy adult at rest, though a blood pressure of 130/80 mmHg is also considered acceptable. (See page 27 for more information about how blood pressure is measured.)

When your heart works harder to pump blood around your body (when you lift a heavy weight or during exercise, for example), it is your systolic pressure that tends to rise. However, as your arteries age and lose their elasticity (as happens in hypertension), it is your diastolic pressure that tends to creep up.

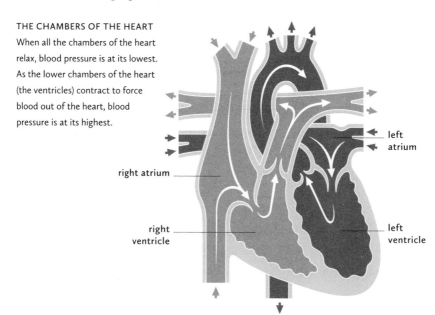

THE CHAMBERS OF THE HEART
When all the chambers of the heart relax, blood pressure is at its lowest. As the lower chambers of the heart (the ventricles) contract to force blood out of the heart, blood pressure is at its highest.

right atrium

right ventricle

left atrium

left ventricle

THE NORMAL CONTROL OF BLOOD PRESSURE

To understand what goes wrong when you have hypertension, it's helpful to know how the healthy body normally regulates blood pressure. These are the main mechanisms:

- Altering the speed and force at which your heart contracts so more or less blood is pumped into your circulation.
- Relaxing or constricting your blood vessels (to vary the amount of blood they hold).
- Regulating the volume of blood in your circulation by altering the amount of salt and fluids filtered out by your kidneys.
- Regulating the volume of blood in your circulation by triggering feelings of thirst, which then prompt you to drink.

These control mechanisms are regulated partly by nerve signals from your central nervous system and partly by hormones and related substances released from various parts of your body, including your kidneys, adrenal glands, pituitary gland, and heart.

BARORECEPTORS: THE BODY'S BLOOD PRESSURE MONITORS

In the walls of your heart and blood vessels are structures called baroreceptors, which help monitor your blood pressure. They work by detecting how stretched your blood vessels are (the greater the pressure your blood exerts on your vessel walls, the more they stretch).

If your blood pressure rises and your blood vessels stretch, your baroreceptors are more highly stimulated than usual. This sets in action a chain of events that causes your blood pressure to fall: your heart rate slows, your blood vessels dilate, and the secretion of blood-vessel constricting chemicals decreases. When your baroreceptors detect a fall in blood pressure (for example, when you go from lying down to a standing position), they trigger an increase in your heart rate. They also trigger the prompt increase of an important hormone called renin (see page 16). Signals constantly pass between your baroreceptors and your brain to keep your blood pressure at a normal level.

THE RENIN-ANGIOTENSIN SYSTEM

Renin is a hormone produced by your kidneys and released into your bloodstream. It sets off a chain reaction that culminates in the rise of your blood pressure. Renin acts ona substance in the blood called angiotensin. As a result, angiotensin I is produced.

Angiotensin I, in turn, is quickly acted upon by angiotensin converting enzyme (ACE) to form angiotensin II. Angiotensin II causes your arteries to constrict rapidly, which raises both your systolic and diastolic blood pressures. Angiotensin II is one of the most powerful blood vessel constrictors known. One of the mainstays of high blood pressure treatment is a group of drugs that block angiotensin converting enzyme. These are known as ACE inhibitors (see page 34). Another type of drug prescribed for hypertension is beta-blockers—among other actions, these lower blood pressure by decreasing the body's secretion of renin.

As well as causing your arteries to constrict, angiotensin II triggers feelings of thirst (drinking increases the volume of fluid in your body and, therefore, your blood pressure). It also increases the secretion of two hormones: antidiuretic hormone and aldosterone. Both of these help raise blood pressure.

THE ROLE OF ANTIDIURETIC HORMONE

Antidiuretic hormone, also known as vasopressin, is released by your brain's pituitary gland when prompted to by angiotensin II. It acts on your kidneys to decrease urine production. This means more fluid stays in your body, which helps to raise your blood pressure.

THE ROLE OF ALDOSTERONE

Aldosterone is a steroid hormone secreted by your adrenal glands. It increases the reabsorption of sodium (in exchange for potassium) from your urine, sweat, saliva, and intestinal juices. This draws fluid back into your body to help increase blood volume and raise blood pressure.

One rare cause of secondary hypertension (the less common type; see pages 20–22) is the excessive production of aldosterone by the adrenal glands. This is known as Conn's syndrome.

LOW BLOOD PRESSURE

Some people have blood pressure that is too low—known medically as hypotension. The symptoms are dizziness and fainting. Hypotension can be caused by heart problems, taking certain drugs, or excessive fluid loss from the body as a result of diarrhea or major bleeding from an injury.

THE ROLE OF NATRIURETIC HORMONE

The other important hormone in blood pressure regulation is natriuretic hormone, which is secreted by the heart. In contrast to the hormones mentioned above, natriuretic hormone lowers blood pressure. It does this by inhibiting the secretion of renin from the kidneys and increasing the excretion of sodium and water. It also inhibits the secretion of antidiuretic hormone from the pituitary gland in the brain.

WHAT IS HYPERTENSION?

Hypertension is the medical term for high blood pressure. If you have hypertension, your blood pressure is high all the time—even when you are at rest. People may wonder if the words "hyper" and "tension" imply a nervous, hyper, or tense personality. The answer is no: "hypertension" refers strictly to elevated blood pressure, rather than temperament.

Although hypertension is usually symptomless, it can pose a serious threat to your long-term health if you don't make changes to your diet and lifestyle, or manage it by taking medication prescribed by your doctor.

For 90 percent of people with high blood pressure, no obvious single cause is identified. They are described as having primary or essential hypertension. For the other 10 percent, an identifiable cause is discovered —these people are referred to as having secondary hypertension.

ESSENTIAL HYPERTENSION

The exact cause of essential hypertension remains unknown, but it's thought to result from an interaction between inherited, developmental, and lifestyle factors.

INHERITED FACTORS

Your genetic makeup influences how well your body is able to control your blood pressure. Genes can affect:

- The sensitivity of your baroreceptors (see page 15) and your renin-angiotensin system (see page 16).
- The responsiveness of your blood vessels to signals that tell them to dilate or constrict.
- How well your kidneys are able to flush excess sodium and fluid from your circulation.
- How an amino acid called homocysteine is processed by your body. Abnormal homocysteine processing results in a blood pressure rise of 0.7/0.5 mmHg in men and 1.2/0.7 mmHg in women for each 0.68 mg/L increase in circulating homocysteine concentrations. If homocysteine builds up, it hastens the development of atherosclerosis (see pages 19–20), contributing to the development of hypertension.

DEVELOPMENTAL FACTORS

An inadequate diet during pregnancy can affect the way the circulatory system forms in the developing embryo. It has been found that low birthweight babies are more likely to develop hypertension as adults. Researchers have found that average adult systolic blood pressure increases by 11 mmHg as birthweight goes down from 7½ pounds to 5½ pounds. The highest blood pressures occur in men and women who were

---

HYPERTENSION AND SCAR TISSUE

An interesting predictor of whether someone will develop hypertension is the way in which their body forms scars. Some people produce an excessive amount of scar tissue in response to injury and have large, lumpy scars. These people are twice as likely to develop hypertension compared with those who produce normal scar tissue. The link between scar tissue and hypertension appears to be angiotensin II (see page 16); as well as raising blood pressure, angiotensin II stimulates production of collagen—the fibrous protein found in scar tissue.

born as small babies with large placentas. Poor nutrition during early development also affects your fingerprint patterns (which form arches, loops, or whorls). Adults with one whorl have a blood pressure that is 6 percent higher than in those with no whorls, and blood pressure increases as the number of whorls increase (the maximum number is ten: two per digit) with most people having two or three.

LIFESTYLE FACTORS

Scientists now know lifestyle factors interact with inherited factors to predispose certain people to hypertension in later life. These lifestyle factors include:

- Smoking cigarettes.
- Consuming excess salt in your diet.
- Drinking too much alcohol.
- Stress.
- Lack of exercise.
- Poor nutrition.
- Following a high-glycemic index diet (see pages 77–78).
- Obesity.
- A low intake of vitamins B6, B12, and folate. (This increases your likelihood of developing hypertension if your ability to process the amino acid homocysteine is poor.)

The good news is that, even if you are genetically or developmentally predisposed to high blood pressure, you can take steps to prevent or delay its onset—this book will show you how.

ATHEROSCLEROSIS

This is the hardening and furring of the arteries that happens naturally with age, but which is hastened by many of the risk factors described above. Atherosclerosis is a main cause of high blood pressure. As arteries lose elasticity, the walls become increasingly hard and rigid. They also "fur up"—fatty deposits, known as atheromas, are laid down on the lining

FURRED-UP ARTERIES

As people get older, their arteries tend to lose flexibility. Not only do arteries become more rigid, they also get furred up with fatty deposits. This is called atherosclerosis and it is both a cause and an effect of hypertension.

HEALTHY ARTERY

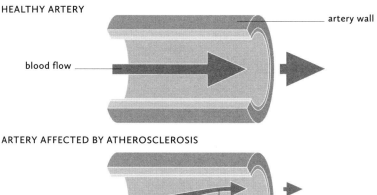

ARTERY AFFECTED BY ATHEROSCLEROSIS

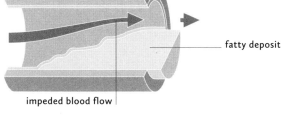

of the artery walls. Hard arteries can no longer dilate effectively, and furred arteries make the flow of blood slower because the diameter of the artery is narrowed. The combined effect is a rise in dystolic blood pressure. Conversely, high blood pressure can also hasten atherosclerosis (see pages 19–20). It does this by putting the artery walls under excessive strain.

SECONDARY HYPERTENSION

Hypertension that has a single major underlying cause is known as secondary hypertension.

KIDNEY DISEASE

In the majority of cases of secondary hypertension, the cause is a kidney (renal) disease that prevents excess fluid and salts being filtered from the body properly. They build up in the circulation and the result is a rise in blood pressure. The kidneys also secrete an increased amount of renin hormone (see page 34), contributing to the development of hypertension.

YOUR HOMOCYSTEINE LEVEL

A raised homocysteine level is linked with damage to the arteries and an increased risk of heart attack and stroke. Make sure you know your homocysteine level—ask your doctor for a test or buy a home test.

PREGNANCY

In five to seven percent of pregnancies, women experience a type of secondary hypertension known as pre-eclampsia. This usually resolves itself after childbirth.

DRUG SIDE-EFFECTS

Some drugs, including some over-the-counter drugs, can cause secondary hypertension. These include nonsteroidal anti-inflammatory drugs (for example, ibuprofen), which can raise blood pressure by 5–10 mmHg; the combined oral contraceptive pill which, after several years' use, increases blood pressure by an average of 2.8/1.9 mmHg; ephedrine (a nasal decongestant); prednisolone (an oral corticosteroid); and monoamine-oxidase inhibitors (an older type of antidepressant that causes sudden rises in blood pressure when eating specific foods); and carbenoxolone (sometimes used to treat stomach ulcers), which encourages the retention of sodium and water.

RARE CAUSES

Although rare, secondary hypertension can be caused by the following:

- Anatomical abnormalities (such as congenital narrowing of the aorta or renal artery).
- Excess production of red blood cells (polycythemia), which increases blood volume and stickiness.
- Excess production of aldosterone hormone (Conn's syndrome).
- Excessive exposure to corticosteroids (Cushing's syndrome).
- Excess production of growth hormone (acromegaly).
- Excess production of parathyroid hormone (hyperparathyroidism).
- A rare type of adrenal gland tumor (pheochromocytoma).

THE SYMPTOMS OF HYPERTENSION

When blood pressure rises temporarily in a healthy person—during exercise, for example—there are few, if any, symptoms (some people feel a pounding in their ears). There is often the same lack of symptoms in hypertension. Symptoms that do occur tend to be nonspecific, such as headache or passing urine more often at night. The latter symptom occurs when hypertension is linked with fluid retention—lying down causes excess fluid to be redistributed and filtered out by the kidneys.

It's only when blood pressure is severely raised that you get more specific symptoms such as dizziness, visual disturbances, or the occasional nosebleed. This is why regular blood pressure checks are so important.

COMPLICATIONS OF HYPERTENSION

Although hypertension is often symptomless, it's vital to treat it, because, unchecked, it can lead to life-threatening illnesses, such as kidney problems, eye disease, coronary heart disease, stroke, and peripheral vascular disease. Even if you don't yet have these complications, you should be aware of them.

KIDNEY PROBLEMS

The role of the kidneys is to filter the blood and to rid your body of waste products in the form of urine. The kidneys also maintain a healthy amount of fluid and salts in your body. In the long term, high blood pressure can lead to the hardening and furring of the arteries that supply the kidneys. It can also damage small blood vessels inside the kidneys. As a result, the kidneys receive a poor supply of blood and they can:

- Start to shrink (atrophy).
- Function less well and produce less urine.
- Leak protein into the urine (this is an important sign of many early kidney diseases).

DAMAGE TO THE KIDNEYS

If the renal artery that supplies the kidneys becomes hard and narrow, the kidneys can be damaged by an inadequate blood supply. High blood pressure in the tiny blood vessels inside the kidney can also damage the kidney's filtering units—the nephrons.

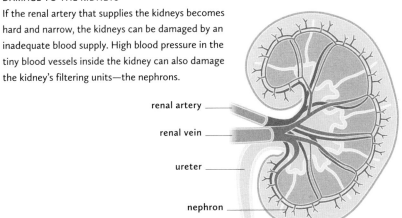

renal artery

renal vein

ureter

nephron

Damage to the kidneys is often symptomless. In fact, by the time you start to experience symptoms—such as swollen ankles, shortness of breath, itchy skin, and nausea—your kidneys have already lost a significant amount of their filtering ability. At this point you will be losing protein into your urine. If damage continues, your kidneys will produce progressively less urine, and waste products and fluid will remain in your body. The late symptoms of kidney disease include swelling of the abdomen, face, and limbs; weight loss; vomiting; and severe lethargy.

Kidney damage is usually diagnosed by a variety of urine and blood tests. At first, kidney damage can be managed by tight control of your blood pressure. You will be prescribed medication to reduce the amount of protein you lose in your urine. During the later stages of kidney damage, treatment can consist of dialysis or a kidney transplant. Dialysis involves artificially filtering your blood, sometimes with a dialysis machine.

EYE DISEASE

Over time, hypertension can damage the small blood vessels in the retinas at the back of the eyes. This is known as hypertensive retinopathy. In the early stages of retinopathy, your vision is unaffected. However, in later stages of retinopathy, your vision can be reduced and, in severe cases, you may have partial or complete sight loss. Hypertension is

DAMAGE TO THE RETINA

The retina is the area at the back of the eye that receives light. Like other blood vessels in the body, the retinal blood vessels are susceptible to damage by hypertension. If the damage is unchecked, this can lead to a loss of vision.

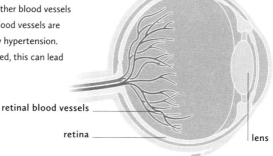

retinal blood vessels

retina

lens

usually diagnosed and treated before it becomes this severe. People with high blood pressure should have regular eye examinations to check for signs of damage to the retina. Retinal changes are divided into the following stages of severity:

• Stage I: the retinal arteries appear thickened and bulging.
• Stage II: the arteries compress the veins where they cross.
• Stage III: the arteries leak blood and fluid.
• Stage IV: the optic nerve swells and bulges.

If stage III retinal changes are diagnosed, your hypertension urgently needs to be controlled. Stage III changes are associated with a similar level of deterioration to the blood vessels in the brain—this puts you at risk of a stroke (see page 19). You might be asked to stay in hospital until your hypertension is under control.

CORONARY HEART DISEASE (CHD)

Over time, high blood pressure can hasten the development of a condition called atherosclerosis (see pages 25–26), in which the arteries become hard and narrowed with fatty deposits known as atheromas. (It can also work the other way around: atherosclerosis can lead to high blood pressure.)

If your coronary arteries are affected by atherosclerosis, the blood flow to your heart is less efficient. As damage progresses, your heart will receive an insufficient supply of oxygen and this can lead to the symptoms of coronary heart disease, which are described below.

Coronary heart disease can be treated with either medicine or surgery. Surgery can include coronary artery bypass surgery or coronary angioplasty. Bypass surgery involves grafting a blood vessel from another part of your body to divert blood away from the damaged section. Angioplasty involves widening the artery by inserting a fine tube into the artery. A balloon on the tip of the tube is inflated inside the blocked section, then deflated and withdrawn. The symptoms of coronary heart disease are as follows:

ANGINA

This refers to a sensation of pain or pressure in your chest that comes and goes. It usually occurs when you are stressed or when you exert yourself. You might also experience pain in your left shoulder or on the inside of your left arm.

HEART ATTACK

This is a sudden pain in the chest that can be accompanied by breathlessness, a pounding heart, sweating, nausea, light-headedness, and sometimes, loss of consciousness. Heart attack symptoms are sometimes relatively mild.

HEART FAILURE

The heart, rather than failing completely as the name of this condition suggests, gradually loses its ability to pump blood around your body. This leads to swelling in your legs, feet, and abdomen; severe tiredness; and breathlessness.

STROKE

If atherosclerosis affects the flow of blood to your brain, you are at risk of a blood clot, or a leakage of blood into the brain (as a result of a burst vessel). If this happens, you have a stroke. Your brain is deprived of oxygen and brain cells in the affected area are damaged or die. The symptoms of a stroke depend on which part of your brain has been damaged. Your vision, speech, memory, hearing, movement, or balance can be affected.

The treatment of a stroke consists of helping you recover the functions that were lost or damaged. For example, you might receive physiotherapy to restore movement or speech therapy to help you talk again.

PERIPHERAL VASCULAR DISEASE

Peripheral vascular disease occurs when the arteries in your legs and arms become narrowed by fatty deposits that restrict the flow of blood. Because blood cannot get through, your leg muscles are prone to cramping, especially during physical activity when their demand for blood and oxygen increases. In severe cases, just walking a short distance on flat ground can cause cramping. In very severe cases, pain can even occur when you are sitting down. Peripheral vascular disease is most likely if you have hypertension and you are a smoker, or if you also have diabetes.

Peripheral vascular disease can also make it difficult for men to achieve or maintain an erection, because narrowed arteries mean blood supply to the penis is reduced.

The treatment for peripheral vascular disease consists of pills or surgery—either bypass surgery or angioplasty; see page 25.

BLOOD SUPPLY TO THE LEGS
The legs need a plentiful supply of blood from the arteries for muscles to work properly. If the flow of blood is restricted, the muscles start to cramp and movement is impeded.

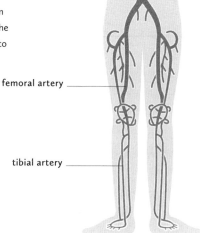

femoral artery

tibial artery

DIAGNOSIS AND SCREENING

Your blood pressure can rise from year to year, which is why it's important to monitor it regularly. As you get older, you should have your blood pressure checked at least once every three years, and preferably annually. Blood pressure is checked using a sphygmomanometer. This consists of a cuff that is attached to a digital blood pressure monitor. The cuff is wrapped around your upper arm and inflated to a high pressure, which stops blood from flowing to your lower arm. As the cuff is slowly deflated, the monitor reads your systolic and diastolic blood pressure (see pages 13–14).

If you're diagnosed with hypertension, you will be described as having prehypertension or stages 1, 2, or 3. It can be possible to treat stage 1 hypertension with lifestyle changes, but stages 2 and 3 are usually treated with medication in combination with lifestyle changes—see pages 30–35 for more about treatment.

WHITE-COAT HYPERTENSION

A doctor usually takes your blood pressure several times before diagnosing hypertension. This is because your blood pressure can be high on one occasion, but not on the next—some people feel so anxious about the experience of visiting the doctor or having their blood pressure taken it causes a rise in their blood pressure. This is known as "white-coat hypertension." White-coat hypertension, which can increase systolic blood pressure by 20–30 mmHg, is suspected when a person has a normal blood pressure when they check it at home, but a high reading in the presence of a doctor.

If there is doubt about a diagnosis of hypertension, a doctor might recommend your blood pressure is monitored over a 24-hour period, using an ambulatory monitoring device. This consists of a cuff that is attached to a monitor by a tube. The cuff, which you wear around your arm for 24 hours, inflates and deflates at intervals to measure your blood pressure.

WHAT YOUR BLOOD PRESSURE READING MEANS

Blood pressure reading	Classification	Treatment
120/80mmHg	Optimal	No treatment necessary (though always adopt a healthy lifestyle).
130/80mmHg	Normal	Reassess in five years and adopt a healthy lifestyle.
130/80–139/89mmHg	Pre-hypertension	Reassess yearly (treat if there is high risk of heart disease).
140/90–159/99mmHg	Stage 1 hypertension (mild)	If no complications, no diabetes and a low risk of cardio-vascular problems, monitor blood pressure every two to three months and reassess risk of cardiovascular disease annually. If complications, diabetes or a high risk of cardiovascular disease, treat with medication. In both cases, make lifestyle changes.
160/100–179/109mmHg*	Stage 2 hypertension (moderate)	Treat with medication and lifestyle changes.
180/110mmHg	Stage 3 hypertension (severe)	Treat with medication and lifestyle changes.

* Or a sustained diastolic blood pressure of equal to or above 100mmHg, despite diet and lifestyle measures.

SCREENING FOR COMPLICATIONS

If you're diagnosed with hypertension, your doctor will want to find out whether you have developed any of the complications associated with high blood pressure (see pages 22–26), such as coronary heart disease or eye disease. For example, he or she may look for signs of excess fluid in your body (this can be a sign of heart failure) by pressing on the skin of your lower limbs to see if this leaves a mark. He or she will also listen to your heart and lungs using a stethoscope. Other tests that may be carried out are:

EYE EXAMINATION

The retinas at the backs of your eyes can be damaged by high blood pressure—this is called hypertensive retinopathy. Your doctor can check for this by looking into your eyes with an ophthalmoscope. The health of the blood vessels in the backs of your eye can provide useful information about the health of your cardiovascular system in general. For example, one 2006 study confirmed having retinopathy is linked with double the risk of heart enlargement and stroke.

URINE TEST

High blood pressure can damage your kidneys. Your urine will be tested for the presence of substances that may indicate kidney damage.

CHEST X-RAY

An x-ray reveals the size and shape of your heart. It can also detect heart failure, which is a symptom of coronary heart disease.

ELECTROCARDIOGRAM (ECG)

This measures the rhythm and electrical activity of your heart. It can show how high blood pressure has affected the working of your heart and whether you have had a heart attack.

BLOOD TESTS

Your blood is tested for levels of fats such as cholesterol and triglycerides—high levels of some fats (see pages 72–73) increase your risk of coronary heart disease. Your blood level of an amino acid called homocysteine is also assessed. High homocysteine promotes atherosclerosis (see pages 19–20) and abnormal blood clotting. As many as one in 10 heart attacks and strokes can be attributable to raised homocysteine, making it at least as important a risk factor as high cholesterol. Your blood will also be tested for glucose and salt (sodium, potassium, and chloride) levels.

INTERPRETING HOMOCYSTEINE LEVELS	
Homocysteine level	Risk level
0.93 mg/l	Optimum (low risk)
0.94–1.34 mg/l	Mild risk
1.35–1.74 mg/l	Medium risk
1.75–2.7 mg/l	High risk
Above 2.7 mg/l	Very high risk

TREATING HYPERTENSION

The early diagnosis and treatment of hypertension is important to reduce the risk of the complications described on pages 22–26. Once your doctor has established you have hypertension, he or she will recommend that you make a number of lifestyle changes. Depending on your stage of hypertension (see page 28), he or she might also prescribe drugs. Blood pressure treatment aims to bring your systolic blood pressure to 140 mmHg or below and your diastolic blood pressure to 90 mmHg or below. If you have coronary heart disease (CHD) or are at high risk of it, a lower target of 130/80 mmHg is recommended.

ADJUSTING YOUR LIFESTYLE

A doctor will encourage you to make the following diet and lifestyle changes. These can help you avoid drug treatment, or they can complement the blood pressure-lowering effects of medication, perhaps enabling you to reduce the dose or number of drugs you need.

- Adults should eat at least 2 cups fruit and 2 cups vegetables per day, depending on their age and gender (see pages 69–72).
- Reduce your intake of unhealthy fat, such as saturated fat (see pages 72–75).

- Healthy children and adults need less than ¼ teaspoon salt a day (see pages 76–77).
- If you smoke, quit (see pages 95–97).
- Limit your alcohol intake to no more than one drink a day for women, or two drinks if you are a man (see pages 97–99).
- Find coping strategies to help you deal with stress.
- Get regular aerobic exercise, such as brisk walking, for at least 30 minutes a day, ideally on most days of the week (see pages 100–102).
- Lose weight if you need to. Then maintain a healthy weight for your height (see pages 102–105).

DRUG TREATMENTS

If your blood pressure is elevated to a level that requires drug treatment, your doctor will select one or more medications from the following classes. These drugs are taken in tablet or capsule form and are known as anti-hypertensives.

- Thiazide diuretics.
- Beta-blockers.
- Calcium channel blockers.
- ACE inhibitors.
- Angiotensin II blockers.
- Renin inhibitors may also become available.

MONITORING HYPERTENSION

When you have hypertension it's important to monitor your blood pressure at home. Selfinflating upper arm and wrist monitors are validated as accurate, though the measurements you obtain are typically lower than those measured by a doctor—probably because you are more relaxed at home. A home measurement of less than 130/80 mmHg is considered optimal. If possible, buy a monitor with a memory so you can record your readings at the same time of day every week. Your doctor can then download the information.

Because hypertension is unlikely to make you feel ill on a day-to-day level, it can be frustrating to have to take pills. However, your medication is a crucial investment in your future health. Together with diet and lifestyle changes, it reduces the risk of life-threatening conditions such as stroke and coronary heart disease.

People often ask how long they must take anti-hypertensives for. Although many people have to take them for life, this is not inevitable. It might be possible to stop taking anti-hypertensives if you don't have any complications of hypertension, and if you successfully lower your blood pressure by adopting the diet and lifestyle measures on pages 30–31. However, it is important once you start taking a drug, that you don't make any changes without consulting your doctor. If your doctor decides you can lower the dose of your medication, or stop taking it all together, he or she will decrease the dose in a gradual stepwise fashion. This is necessary to avoid a sudden increase in your blood pressure.

In my opinion, the way to get the best from anti-hypertensive drugs is to take a close interest in your blood pressure (see the box on page 31 on monitoring hypertension). If you notice that your blood pressure isn't responding to a new drug, or an increase in the dose of a drug, ask your doctor to review your treatment. On the other hand, if your home monitoring reveals that your blood pressure is coming down (thanks to losing weight, for example), ask your doctor about lowering your dose.

SECONDARY HYPERTENSION

If you are thought to have secondary hypertension (the less common type of hypertension), you'll be tested for the possible underlying causes and these will be treated appropriately. Your blood will be tested for levels of hormones that control blood pressure, such as aldosterone, cortisol, and renin. Your blood or urine will also be assessed for levels of substances that, if raised, are known to cause hypertension. For example, a high level of vanillylmandelic acid can indicate a tumor of the adrenal glands. You will also have an ultrasound scan of the kidneys or other kidney tests—this is because kidney disease is the most common underlying cause of secondary hypertension.

THIAZIDE DIURETICS

Thiazide diuretics lower your blood pressure by increasing the loss of salts and fluid through your urine. They typically act within one to two hours of taking them. For this reason it is better to take them in the morning rather than at night so you won't need to get out of bed to empty your bladder.

At first, you might notice you are urinating more often than usual. This wears off after the first few days because thiazides also encourage the mild dilation of small arteries so fluid in your circulation is redistributed. High doses of thiazides are avoided as they can lead to sodium/potassium imbalances. Thiazide diuretics are often prescribed to older people who also have heart failure. They are not prescribed if you have gout, as they can aggravate this condition.

BETA-BLOCKERS

Beta-blockers lower blood pressure in the following ways:

- Decreasing the workload of your heart by slowing your pulse to about 60 beats per minute and reducing the force of each heartbeat.
- Reducing the sensitivity of baroreceptors (blood pressure sensors in the walls of your heart and blood vessels; see page 15).
- Altering the way blood vessels dilate or constrict.
- Blocking the effects of the stress hormone adrenaline.
- Lowering the secretion of a kidney hormone, renin (see page 16).

If beta-blockers need to be stopped, the dose is usually tapered off gradually so your blood pressure does not suddenly increase (known as rebound hypertension). Beta-blockers are best avoided in people with asthma, as they can trigger an attack. Their most troublesome side-effects include fatigue, cold extremities, and problems with sexual function. A beta-blocker is ideal for someone with angina or who has previously had a heart attack. However, in general there is a move away from using beta-blockers for hypertension.

CALCIUM CHANNEL BLOCKERS

Calcium channel blockers slow the movement of calcium into your muscle cells. This reduces the force of contraction of the heart, relaxes arteries, reduces arterial spasm, and allows peripheral veins to dilate so they hold more blood. Side-effects can include flushing, headache, ankle swelling, and constipation. A calcium channel blocker is often selected for older people who have a raised systolic blood pressure, but a relatively normal diastolic blood pressure, or who have angina. Some doctors favor a move toward using calcium channel blockers (and ACE inhibitors) as a first-line treatment option in preference to thiazide diuretics or beta-blockers.

ACE INHIBITORS

One of the body's most powerful ways of increasing blood pressure is the renin-angiotensin system (see page 16), which involves angiotensin-converting enzyme (ACE). Drugs that block the action of this enzyme (ACE inhibitors) prevent the production of angiotensin II—a powerful blood vessel constrictor. Small arteries and veins are, therefore, able to dilate, causing blood pressure to fall. By increasing blood flow to your kidneys, this class of drug also encourages the loss of water and sodium in your urine.

Because ACE inhibitors can cause a sudden fall in blood pressure with the very first dose, treatment is often started at night when going to bed. One of the most troublesome side-effects of the drug is a persistent dry cough. An ACE inhibitor is often selected for people who also have heart pump failure. Some doctors favor a general move toward using ACE inhibitors (and calcium channel blockers) as a first-line treatment option in preference to thiazide diuretics or beta-blockers.

ANGIOTENSIN II BLOCKERS

Angiotensin II blockers are similar to ACE inhibitors, but they work one step farther, in that they block the formation of angiotensin II (see page 16). The end result is the same: dilation of arteries and veins, increased blood flow to the kidneys and increased production of urine. Interestingly, angiotensin II blockers can also act on the central nervous system to

HOW DRUGS ARE PRESCRIBED

Your doctor will select the most appropriate drug for you depending on your age and whether you have complications.

The lowest recommended dose of the drug is prescribed.

This often produces an effect within 24 hours, but your full response to the drug is monitored over at least four weeks (unless your blood pressure needs lowering urgently).

After four weeks the dose of the drug is slowly increased according to the manufacturer's instructions..

If the increase doesn't adequately control your blood pressure, a second or third drug is added.

If your blood pressure remains too high, another drug is added.

reduce thirst so you drink less. Side-effects of these drugs, such as dizziness, are usually mild.

OTHER ANTI-HYPERTENSIVE DRUGS

Some other anti-hypertensive drugs are used in special cases, such as pregnancy. In addition, another group of drugs called alpha-blockers (for example, Doxazosin, Prazosin, and Terazosin) are mainly reserved for use in men who have urinary symptoms due to an enlarged prostate gland—alpha-blockers help shrink the prostate gland as well as reducing blood pressure.

ADDITIONAL DRUGS THAT MIGHT BE PRESCRIBED

In addition to anti-hypertensive drugs, your doctor may also prescribe other drugs. These could include statin drugs, which lower the level of unhealthy cholesterol in your blood (as with hypertension, high cholesterol is a risk factor for cardiovascular disease). Aspirin is also sometimes prescribed because of its ability to prevent abnormal blood clotting.

PART TWO
THE NATURAL HEALTH APPROACH

In this chapter I explain how you can lower your blood pressure using complementary therapies, and making dietary and lifestyle changes. These tools can not only lower your blood pressure, but can also improve your overall health and well-being. In many cases, these natural approaches to treatment work so well your doctor might wish to reduce the number or dose of drugs you're taking. The complementary therapies in this chapter are safe and effective for people with hypertension—some, such as aromatherapy, reflexology, and yoga, can lower blood pressure by relaxing you, while others, such as acupressure, acupuncture, and herbal medicine, work on a deeper level. Perhaps one of the most exciting approaches is that of dietary change: relatively simple steps such as cutting back on your salt intake; consuming more fruit, vegetables, fish, and garlic; eating superfoods, such as almonds; and even enjoying small amounts of red wine and dark chocolate have the power to transform your health. Key nutritional supplements can also have a positive impact on your blood pressure. Finally, I look at how changing your lifestyle will help you. Getting more exercise, maintaining a healthy weight, not smoking, enjoying alcohol in moderation, and reducing stress can literally add years to your life.

COMPLEMENTARY APPROACHES TO TREATMENT

The holistic approach to treating hypertension includes a number of complementary therapies you can use in conjunction with any medicines your doctor prescribes. In many cases, you will benefit from visiting a therapist, at least at first.

If you have pre-hypertension or stage I hypertension (see pages 17–18) and are not yet taking medication, it's likely complementary approaches, together with dietary and lifestyle changes, will lower your blood pressure to a point where you won't need drugs. If you're already taking medication to treat hypertension, it is important to continue taking your drugs alongside any therapies you try. That's why therapies are best referred to as complementary, rather than alternative, therapies—they *complement* medical treatment, rather than providing a true alternative. Another phrase used to describe the combined use of orthodox and complementary therapies is "integrative medicine," which, essentially, cherry-picks the best approaches from a number of different philosophies.

WHICH THERAPIES CAN HELP?
Over the next few pages, I give an overview of the main complementary therapies that can help hypertension: aromatherapy, naturopathy, herbal medicine, homeopathy, reflexology, acupuncture, yoga, qigong, and meditation. Some approaches, such as aromatherapy, yoga, and meditation, work mainly through relaxation and overcoming stress, while others, such as homeopathy, reflexology, and acupuncture, harness your body's natural healing abilities to lower your blood pressure. In contrast, herbal medicine uses plant extracts that have a physiological effect in the body, modifying its function in a similar way to some drugs.

CONSULTING A THERAPIST
It is important to consult a qualified practitioner, who is accredited with the appropriate umbrella organization, and who carries indemnity insurance. Most umbrella organizations provide lists of qualified

practitioners who are registered with them. Many also have a facility on their website to help you find a therapist in your area. Some useful addresses are provided in the resource section on page 237.

Having checked the qualifications of your chosen therapist, ask about their experience and successes in treating hypertension. Find out how long a course of treatment is likely to last, and the likely cost, before committing yourself to an appointment. Be sure to check your insurance or HMO policy will cover the treatment before you begin.

Having consulted a therapist, you might find you need only one or two consultations—for example, with a homeopath or medical herbalist—to point you in the right direction and enable you to use that therapy at home. With other therapies, such as reflexology, yoga, and aromatherapy massage, you might decide to attend regularly for on-going practitioner-led benefits.

Always tell the therapist you have hypertension and which, if any, prescribed medications you're taking. If your blood pressure starts coming down as a result of a therapy, tell your doctor.

AROMATHERAPY

The main principle of aromatherapy is that inhaling specific scents can change your physiological state. This happens because smell has an important impact on your brain—in particular, on a primitive part of your brain called the limbic system that helps regulate memory, arousal, emotions, and hormone secretion. The scents used by aromatherapists are essential oils derived from plants. Depending on the particular plant, the essential oil can be harvested from the flowers, leaves, seeds, roots, fruits, or wood.

Essential oils are highly concentrated plant extracts and should be used with care (see the guidelines on page 40). They are almost always diluted with a "carrier" oil, such as avocado, almond, calendula, grapeseed, jojoba, or wheatgerm oil, before use. Dilution is important because neat essential oils can irritate the skin and can have adverse

GUIDELINES FOR USING ESSENTIAL OILS

- Do not take essential oils internally.
- Before using an essential oil blend on your skin, put a small amount on a patch of skin and leave it for an hour to insure you are not sensitive to it.
- Do not use essential oils if you are pregnant, or likely to be, except under specialist advice from an aromatherapist.
- Keep essential oils away from your face and eyes.
- If you are taking homeopathic remedies, do not use peppermint, rosemary, or lavender essential oils as they can neutralize the homeopathic effect.
- Essential oils are flammable, so do not put them on an open flame.
- Avoid thyme, clove, and cinnamon essential oils, which can raise blood pressure.
- Always keep essential oils out of the reach of children.

effects—some can even raise blood pressure. One of the few exceptions to the dilution rule is lavender essential oil, which is often used neat. It's also acceptable to use essential oils neat when you're not applying them to the skin, for example, when adding them to a candlelit diffuser to produce a therapeutic atmosphere.

In the case of hypertension, essential oils can help by relaxing you, promoting sleep, and making you less anxious—all of which help lower your blood pressure. Some essential oils lower blood pressure in other ways, for example, by having a diuretic action on the body, which means they flush out excess fluids.

OILS FOR TREATING HYPERTENSION

If you visit an aromatherapist, he or she will assess your health and choose a blend of essential oils suited to your particular needs. He or she will probably massage the diluted oils into your skin and you might be given an ointment or lotion, or essential oil blend, to take home with you. Your aromatherapist will give you specific instructions about how to use any essential oil product. For more information about consulting an aromatherapist, see page 237.

You can also use aromatherapy as a self-help treatment at home. I suggest you select one, two, three, or four essential oils from the chart on page 42. Base your choice on both the therapeutic effects of the oils and your personal scent preferences. If you choose a scent you really like, you'll relax more easily. How you blend the oils together is also a matter of personal choice. Experiment until you find a scent blend you particularly like. If a blend isn't quite to your liking, add more drops of one or more of the oils—or introduce another you think might be missing. Keep a note of the total number of drops you use so you can dilute it with the correct amount of carrier oil and recreate it again in the future. You can add an essential oil blend to a bath, massage it into your skin, or simply diffuse it in the atmosphere.

When buying essential oils, look for the words "pure essential oil" on the label, rather than "aromatherapy oil." Products with the latter label might contain only small amounts of essential oils and will not have the same therapeutic effect.

AROMATHERAPY BATHS

Select a blend of up to three essential oils. Add 5 drops of the blend to 10 ml of a carrier oil and mix. Run your bath so it's a comfortable temperature, then add the aromatic oil mix once the faucets are turned off. Close the bathroom door to keep in the vapors and soak in the bath 15 to 20 minutes, preferably in candlelight. Lie back comfortably and close your eyes. Allow the scent to fill your entire body and imagine it coursing through your blood vessels, bringing deep relaxation, and lowering your blood pressure. At the end of your bath, dip a wet sponge in the oil mix on the surface of the water and use it to gently massage your whole body before rinsing.

MASSAGE

An oil blend intended to come into contact with your skin for massage should contain a maximum total of 1 drop of essential oil per 24 drops of carrier oil. You can massage parts of your body, such as your legs and feet, by yourself. Smooth the oil blend into your skin using firm stroking movements and then massage large muscles such as your thighs with deep kneading strokes. For difficult-to-reach parts of your body, such as your back, take it in turns with a friend or partner to give a relaxing aromatherapy massage.

ESSENTIAL OILS THAT CAN HELP HYPERTENSION

Relaxing and calming oils	Camomile, cedarwood, clary sage, geranium, jasmine, juniper berry, lavender, lemon, lemongrass, melissa, neroli, orange, petitgrain, rose, sandalwood, ylang-ylang
Oils to promote sleep	Camomile, clary sage, geranium, juniper berry, lavender, lemongrass, melissa, neroli, orange, petitgrain, rose, sandalwood, ylang-ylang
Diuretic oils for hypertension with fluid retention	Camomile, cedarwood, geranium, juniper berry, lemon, peppermint, pine
Oils to help essential hypertension	Clary sage, lavender, lemon, marjoram, melissa

OIL BURNERS

Using an oil burner is a good way to administer essential oils at nighttime to help you sleep. Add 2 or 3 drops of a relaxing blend (for example, lavender or lemongrass blended with neroli) to a little warm water over a burner. Let the relaxing oils diffuse into your bedroom before retiring (make sure the candle is snuffed out before you get into bed). Alternatively, add 2 or 3 drops to a tissue and tuck it under your pillow. Another technique, which I recommend for daytime, is to add a few drops of essential oil to a cotton ball. Place this in a small sealed vial or plastic box, then open and inhale it at intervals throughout the day.

NATUROPATHY

Naturopathy is based on the belief the body can find its own healthy equilibrium given the right conditions, such as a healthy diet, plenty of sleep, regular exercise and relaxation, fresh air, a clean environment, a stress-free lifestyle, plus a positive mental attitude.

A naturopath will work with you to help you reach this state of healthy equilibrium. He or she will use a variety of approaches, including dietary changes, supplements, biochemic tissue salts, herbal remedies, homeopathy, hydrotherapy, massage, reflexology, relaxation techniques (including yoga), and, sometimes, physical manipulation. Many naturopaths are trained in iridology (a system of diagnosis involving examin-ation of the iris of the eye), kinesiology (a system of diagnosis based on muscle strength), hypnotherapy, osteopathy, chiropractic, or psychotherapy. Skin brushing, water sprays, or friction rubs are often used to stimulate skin function and to boost the circulation.

THE IMPORTANCE OF DIET

Naturopathic dietary approaches involve following a wholefood, high fiber—and preferably organic—diet that concentrates on fresh and, preferably, raw foods. A naturopathic diet is ideal for someone with hypertension as it's low in salt and fat, high in fiber and antioxidants, and contains plenty of fruits, vegetables, nuts, seeds, wholegrains, and legumes. For hypertension, garlic and onions are recommended, together with foods rich in potassium, calcium, and magnesium (alfalfa, avocados, broccoli, carrots, celery, lima beans, mushrooms, spinach, and most fruits). Mineral water (eight glasses a day) is crucial to eliminate wastes, and a naturopath will usually advise you to avoid caffeine. Supplements of antioxidants (vitamins C and E), magnesium, potassium, coenzyme Q10, and omega-3 fish oil might be recommended, as well as herbal remedies.

BIOCHEMIC TISSUE SALTS

Naturopaths also use homeopathic remedies based on inorganic salts.

DAILY NATUROPATHIC EXERCISES

Breathe slowly and deeply, so air enters the bottom of your lungs, for two minutes twice a day. Before your daily bath or shower, brush your skin with a loofah or skin brush to improve circulation.

These are known as biochemic tissue salts and are considered vital for health—depletion of any particular salt causes illness. Although biochemic tissue salts are prepared in the same way as homeopathic remedies, their use is very different; whereas the usual principle of homeopathy is "like treats like," tissue salts are given to correct a mineral deficiency. You might be prescribed calcium fluoride for hypertension, or potassium phosphate to relieve stress.

SLEEP AND MENTAL WELL-BEING

Naturopathy emphasizes the importance of sleep. Research suggests a lack of sleep increases activity in the sympathetic nervous system, which can increase blood pressure and pulse rate. Stress reduction is also important. In a study of people with mild to moderate hypertension, 70 percent of those who practiced relaxation reduced their medication after six weeks, and within a year, 55 percent required no medication.

Naturopaths also place great importance on a positive state of mind to help overcome ill health. Interesting research shows that smiling boosts immunity. And hugging family and friends has been shown to produce warm feelings due to release of the hormone oxytocin, which is involved in bonding. Oxytocin has been shown to lower blood pressure by slowing the heart rate at times of stress, especially in women.

HERBAL MEDICINE

Herbal medicine is one of the most ancient complementary therapies. In fact, more than 30 percent of medically prescribed drugs are derived from traditional plant remedies, such as aspirin (from the willow tree and meadowsweet plant), morphine (from opium poppy), and digoxin (from foxglove).

Whereas prescribed drugs contain a single active ingredient that is often manufactured synthetically, herbal supplements contain a blend of natural constituents that have evolved together in synergistic balance. This tends to produce a gentler action with less risk of side-effects.

MAKING A HERBAL INFUSION

Infusions are made in a similar way to tea. Take a handful of the freshly picked herb (mint or lemon balm, for example) and place it in a warm glass or china teapot. Cover with boiling water and leave to infuse for 10 minutes, then strain into a mug and drink.

Different parts of different plants are used to create herbal medicines—roots, flowers, leaves, bark, fruit, or seeds—depending on which has the highest concentration of active ingredients. The relevant part of the plant is usually harvested and made into an infusion (also known as a tea or tisane). Plants can also be dried and ground to produce a powder. This powder can be made into an infusion, an alcohol solution (also known as a tincture), or tablets/capsules. Modern technology also allows the extraction of active ingredients to produce more concentrated remedies.

HERBS FOR TREATING HYPERTENSION

A wide range of herbal remedies are effective for treating hypertension and associated problems, such as atherosclerosis. If you consult a medical herbalist, you might be prescribed one of the herbs I describe on the right. You can also buy or make your own herbal remedies. If I provide dosage information about one of the following herbs, the herb is safe to take without supervision. However, please read the warning in the caution box on page 46 before taking any herbal remedies.

GARLIC (ALLIUM SATIVUM)

Garlic is one of the most effective herbal remedies for people with hypertension. Research shows that it can reduce the risk of heart disease and stroke by 50 percent. It provides a number of beneficial substances, including allicin (diallyl thiosulphinate), ajoene, methylallyl trisulphide and dimethyl trisulphide. It has been found to reduce levels of cholesterol and triglycerides (see page 72) in the blood by about 12 percent after four months of taking it. Garlic also decreases blood stickiness, which makes the formation of clots less likely (hypertension is linked with an increased risk of blood-clotting and stroke).

WHEN TO AVOID TAKING HERBS
Do not take herbal remedies during pregnancy or when breastfeeding, unless you're specifically advised to by a medical herbalist or doctor. If you're taking any prescribed drugs, consult a qualified herbalist or pharmacist before taking a herbal remedy.

Other research shows garlic can also lower blood pressure by dilating small arteries and veins by 4–6 percent, and by improving the elasticity of major arteries. These changes mean the heart has to work less hard to pump blood into the circulation. Garlic has even been shown to reverse atherosclerosis (see pages 19–20) by decreasing the volume of fatty deposits on artery walls. In one study lasting four years, the volume of fatty deposits in the arteries was found to decrease by 15.6 percent in people taking garlic tablets, while people taking an inactive placebo experienced a 2.6 percent increase in the volume of fatty deposits.

In combination, all of these beneficial effects can lower resistance in your arteries so your blood pressure falls. A daily dose of 600–900 mg garlic can reduce systolic blood pressure by an average of 8 percent (and by up to 17 percent) and reduce diastolic blood pressure by an average of 12 percent (and up to 16 percent) within two to three months of treatment. Include garlic in your diet as much as possible (add it near the end of cooking for maximum benefit). Consider taking a daily garlic tablet, too. *Dose:* Select tablets standardized to provide 1000 to 1500 mcg allicin daily.

HAWTHORN (*CRATAEGUS OXYCANTHA AND CRATAEGUS MONOGYNA*)
Hawthorn flowers and berries can lower blood pressure by relaxing the blood vessels in the peripheral circulation and improving blood flow to the heart by dilating the coronary arteries. They also block the action of angiotensin-converting enzyme in a similar way to ACE inhibitor drugs (see page 34). Other benefits include lowering blood pressure by flushing excess fluid and sodium from the circulation. Hawthorn also has a calming effect that helps counteract stress, and it increases the strength and efficiency of the heart's pumping action in people with heart failure (see page 25). Only take hawthorn under the supervision of a medical herbalist.

DANDELION (*TARAXACUM OFFICINALIS*)

Dandelion is good for hypertension linked to water retention. It has a diuretic action that helps to flush excess water and sodium from the body through the kidneys—but only in people with fluid retention. If your water balance is normal, dandelion does not have a diuretic action. *Dose:* 500 mg extracts twice a day. Do not take dandelion if you have active gallstones or obstructive jaundice.

LEMON BALM (*MELISSA OFFICINALIS*)

Lemon balm leaves are used during stressful times for their calming properties. Known as the "scholar's herb," lemon balm is widely recommended for exam stress. Herbalists use it to improve heart function and lower blood pressure. Try drinking tea containing lemon balm for its soothing effects. *Dose:* 650 mg three times a day.

BILBERRY (*VACCINIUM MYRTILLUS*)

Bilberries contain purple antioxidant pigments called anthocyanidins that have been shown to strengthen small blood vessels, especially in the eye. One of the complications of high blood pressure is a deterioration in eyesight caused by retinopathy (see pages 23–24). In some cases, taking bilberry extracts can improve visual acuity by 80 percent within two weeks.

Blueberries provide similar anthocyanidins to bilberries, but in smaller concentrations (as their flesh is cream-colored rather than purple), but it's still worth including blueberries and their juice in your diet. *Dose:* 80–160 mg bilberry extract, three times daily.

ARTICHOKE (*CYNARA SCOLYMUS*)

Unhealthily high cholesterol levels often accompany hypertension and contribute to the development of cardiovascular problems. Artichoke extracts reduce cholesterol levels by decreasing the synthesis of cholesterol in the liver, and by increasing the conversion of cholesterol to bile acids. *Dose:* 320 mg capsules, one to six daily with food.

KUDZU (*PUERARIA LOBATA*)

Also known as Japanese arrowroot, kudzu is a rich source of isoflavone plant hormones. Studies suggest drinking kudzu root tea daily can have a significant impact on hypertension. Kudzu can also be used to help you reduce your alcohol intake. *Dose:* 150 mg three times a day.

BUGLEWEED (*LYCOPUS EUROPAEUS*)

Bugleweed is used to treat heart failure (a complication of hypertension). The aerial parts of the plant increase the contracting power of the heart, dilate blood vessels, reduce heart rate, and have a diuretic action. Take bugleweed only under the supervision of a medical herbalist.

CHRYSANTHEMUM (*CHRYSANTHEMUM MORIFOLIUM*)

Flowers from this species of chrysanthemum are used in traditional Chinese medicine to improve coronary circulation, to increase the pumping action of the heart, and to reduce and stabilize hypertension. Take chrysanthemum only under the supervision of a medical herbalist.

LIME BLOSSOM (*TILIA EUROPEA*)

This is used medicinally to lower blood pressure and promote relaxation.

STANDARDIZATION OF HERBAL PRODUCTS

During the production of commercial herbal remedies, a small sample from each batch is taken.

The amount of one or two important active ingredients in the sample is measured.

The batch is then either diluted or concentrated so a standard amount of active ingredient is present in the finished product.

If you choose a "standardized" herbal product, you can be sure you will receive a consistently effective dose. Standardized remedies are also more likely to have clinical trials supporting their use.

It contains antioxidant flavonoids, plus a natural sedative that relieves tension and promotes sleep. Drink an infusion of lime blossom in the evening before bedtime (you can make your own infusion or buy herbal teabags that blend lime blossom with other beneficial herbs).

MISTLETOE (VISCUM ALBUM)
Mistletoe is used by herbalists to regulate blood pressure in both hypertension and hypotension. It's often combined with hawthorn (see page 46) in the treatment of hypertension. Take it only under the supervision of a medical herbalist.

MOTHERWORT (LEONURUS CARDIACA)
Leaves from the motherwort plant can strengthen the heart muscle, reduce palpitations, regulate a rapid pulse rate, and lower hypertension. Take it only under the supervision of a medical herbalist.

VALERIAN (VALERIANA OFFICINALIS)
Valerian contains natural sedatives that make it one of the most relaxing herbs available. In one trial its sedative effects were almost as strong as a prescription tranquillizer. It's widely used to relieve anxiety, reduce stress, induce sleep, and lower blood pressure, especially when high blood pressure is linked to excessive stress. Try drinking teas containing valerian for its soothing effects. *Dose:* 250–800 mg, two to three times daily. Select products that are standardized to provide at least 0.8 percent valeric acid.

HOMEOPATHY

Homeopathy was founded about 200 years ago by the German physician Samuel Christian Hahnemann (1755–1843). It's based on the belief that tiny amounts of natural substances can stimulate the body's own healing powers. The term "homeopathy" literally means "similar suffering," and natural substances are selected that, if used at full strength, will trigger the same symptoms they are designed to treat. In minuscule homeopathic doses, however, the opposite effect occurs, and symptoms improve. This is the first prin-ciple of homeopathy: like cures like.

The second major principle of homeopathy is that less cures more. This describes the observation that increasing the dilution of a solution increases its potency. So, by diluting noxious substances many millions of times, their healing properties are enhanced and their undesirable side-effects are lost.

How homeopathy works is not completely understood, but contact with the original remedy is believed to polarize water molecules so they retain a unique electromagnetic signature. This is thought to have a dynamic action that boosts your body's own healing power.

HOMEOPATHIC TREATMENTS

Homeopathic remedies are made from plant, animal, or mineral extracts that are chopped or ground, then steeped and shaken in an alcohol/water solution for two to four weeks. This mixture is strained into a dark glass bottle to produce the concentrated mother tincture, from which dilutions are made.

Homeopathic pills are made by adding a few drops of these solutions to lactose (milk sugar) pillules and swirled together. The lactose pills are stored in airtight, dark glass bottles, out of direct sunlight. Take homeopathic remedies in the following way:

- Tip the pill into your mouth from the lid of the bottle or from a spoon (don't handle it).
- Suck or chew the pill—don't swallow it whole.
- Don't eat or drink for 30 minutes before or after taking a remedy.
- Avoid strong tea or coffee, or powerful essential oils, such as rosemary and peppermint. These can diminish the effect of homeopathic remedies.
- If symptoms worsen initially, persevere. This is a sign the remedy is working.
- If there is no improvement, let your homeopath know—you might need a different remedy.

HOMEOPATHIC REMEDIES FOR HYPERTENSION

REMEDY	PREPARED FROM	USED TO TREAT
Baryta carbonicum	Barium carbonate crystals	Headaches; cardiovascular problems, including hypertension
Baryta muriaticum	Barium chloride crystals	Hypertension with a high systolic and low diastolic pressure
Adrenalinum	Adrenaline (epinephrine) hormone	Sustained stress
Glonoinum	Glyceryl trinitrate	Hypertension associated with increased blood flow to the head
Serum anguillar icthyotoxin	Eel serum	Hypertension associated with fluid retention and kidney problems
Thyroidinum	Dried sheep/calf thyroid gland	Hypertension associated with being overweight
Nuxvomica	Strychnine-containing seeds of the poison nut	Intermittent arterial hypertension; stress associated with overwork and lifestyle excesses (smoking, eating or drinking too much)
Crataegus	Hawthorn	Hypertension, irregular pulse or heart failure (gives heart and circulatory support)
Passiflora incarnata	Passionflower	Stress (it calms and soothes the nervous system)
Picric acidum	Picric acid	Headaches; stress due to overwork; fatigue; fluid retention
Phosphoricum acidum	Phosphoric acid	Listlessness; stress due to bad news; lethargy
Ignatia	Seeds from St Ignatius' bean tree	Headache; stress following emotional upset
Arnica montana	Sneezewort	Emotional shock; abnormal blood clotting

HOW EFFECTIVE IS HOMEOPATHY?

Clinical trials show that homeopathy is significantly better than a placebo in treating many chronic conditions, including hayfever, asthma, migraine, skin problems, and rheumatoid arthritis. Some research shows two homeopathic remedies, Baryta carbonicum and Crataegus, can lower systolic and diastolic blood pressure in some people, though results from other studies were less convincing. Homeopathy seems to work best for those with early or borderline hypertension, who are not yet taking medication, or who are on only one anti-hypertensive drug.

CONSULTING A HOMEOPATH

Although you can buy your own homeopathic remedies, I advise visiting a homeopath for treatment that is individually tailored. A homeopath will select your treatment based not just on your symptoms, but also on your constitution, personality, lifestyle, family background, and tastes. For more information about consulting a homeopath, see page 237.

After completing a course of homeopathy, you will usually feel better in yourself with a greatly improved sense of well-being that allows you to cope in a generally more positive way.

REFLEXOLOGY

Reflexology is believed to have originated in India, China, and Egypt, and dates back more than 5,000 years. It was first practiced in the West by Dr. William Fitzgerald in 1913 (he called his technique "zone therapy"). His work was developed further in the 1930s by Eunice Ingham to create what we now know as reflexology. Reflexology relaxes the body, mind, and spirit, improves circulation, and normalizes bodily functions. Its aim is to treat the symptoms and causes of illness.

According to reflexology theory, points on the feet and hands—known as reflexes—relate to internal organs, structures, and their function. These reflexes are represented as maps on the surfaces of the feet and the hands (though most reflexologists work on the feet). The right foot corresponds to the right side of the body, and the left foot to the left side of the body. Reflexes are present all over the foot—on the soles, upper foot, toes, and ankles.

HOW EFFECTIVE IS REFLEXOLOGY?

Reflexology is said to work best for disorders of the internal organs and for stress-related problems such as headache. A survey carried out in the UK found that stress and hypertension were the conditions most successfully treated by reflexology.

REFLEXES ON THE SOLES OF THE FEET
These are simplified reflexology diagrams showing some of the foot reflexes that correspond with major body organs. If you have hypertension, a reflexologist is likely to work on your heart, thyroid, spine, and kidney reflexes. He or she might also work on your chest reflexes, which are on the top of your feet.

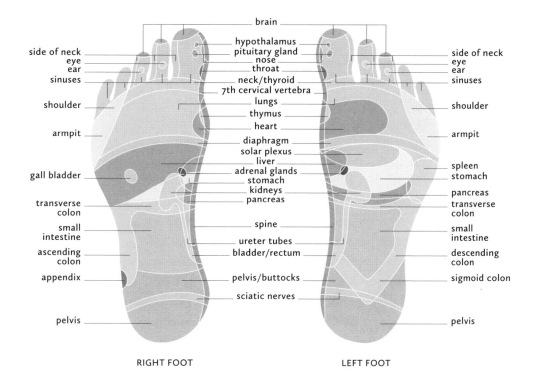

brain
hypothalamus
pituitary gland
nose
throat
neck/thyroid
7th cervical vertebra
lungs
thymus
heart
diaphragm
solar plexus
liver
adrenal glands
stomach
kidneys
pancreas
spine
ureter tubes
bladder/rectum
pelvis/buttocks
sciatic nerves

side of neck
eye
ear
sinuses

shoulder

armpit

gall bladder

transverse
colon

small
intestine

ascending
colon

appendix

pelvis

side of neck
eye
ear
sinuses

shoulder

armpit

spleen
stomach

pancreas

transverse
colon

small
intestine

descending
colon

sigmoid colon

pelvis

RIGHT FOOT   LEFT FOOT

SELF-HELP REFLEXOLOGY

Although I recommend consulting a reflexologist for professional and individually tailored treatment, you can also benefit from massaging the reflexes in your feet yourself. To do this, familiarize yourself with the position of the diaphragm line, which stretches across the ball of each foot. The following massage will take a total of 10 minutes. Try to do it on at least two days a week, morning and evening —or on a daily basis, if you wish.

1 Sit comfortably in a chair. Take a few moments to relax and center yourself. Take some deep breaths and make your exhalations long and smooth. Bring your left foot up on to your right thigh.

2 Using your thumb, gently massage the heart and lung reflexes, which lie between the diaphragm line and the base of your toes. Do this for one minute.

3 Now massage the heart area, which lies between the diaphragm line and the base of your big toe (this area is bigger on the left foot than on the right, because the left ventricle has thicker walls than the right ventricle). Do this for one minute.

4 Massage across the diaphragm line for one minute.

5 Massage along the spinal reflex, which runs along the inner edge of each foot from the top of the big toe to the side of the heel. Do this for one minute.

6 Finally, massage inside the arch of your foot, which contains reflexes relating to your left kidney and adrenal gland. Do this for one minute.

7 Repeat the massage on your right foot.

CONSULTING A REFLEXOLOGIST

A therapist massages your feet using firm thumb and finger pressure. He or she also treats specific problems by applying pressure to appropriate reflex points. This stimulates nerve endings that pass from your feet to your brain and then to the relevant part of your body.

While massaging your feet, a therapist might also come across points on your feet that are unusually tender. By observing which bodily organs these points are related to, it's possible to diagnose health problems you might not be aware of. A reflexologist can treat these problems by working on the tender spots.

To treat hypertension, a reflexologist will typically concentrate on your heart reflex, which stretches from the diaphragm line (see diagram on page 53) toward the base of the toes on both feet. Massaging the heart reflex on your left foot is said to strengthen and regulate your heart, while concentrating on the diaphragm line helps deepen your breathing and bring more oxygen into your body.

On the sole of your foot, at the base of your big toes, is the reflex area for the thyroid and parathyroid glands. Stimulating these helps to regulate your pulse rate and calcium metabolism, which can have a positive effect on your blood pressure. Finally, your spinal reflex, on the inside edge of both feet, is massaged to support your nervous system. Massaging the kidney areas (located at the top of your arches) helps flush excess fluid from your body. At the end of each session, you should feel warm, contented, and relaxed.

ACUPUNCTURE

Acupuncture is part of traditional Chinese medicine (TCM). It's based on the belief we all have a vibrant life energy, known as qi or chi (pronounced "chee") flowing through our body along specific channels known as meridians. There are 12 major meridians, that correspond to organs in the body. Qi enters the meridians from outside the body, flows in a specific direction along the meridians and nourishes our internal organs in the process. As long as qi energy flows smoothly along the meridians, we live in a state of health and balance. But if the flow of qi is disrupted by factors such as stress, poor diet, and spiritual neglect, there will be an imbalance in energy flow. This results in the symptoms of ill health. According to traditional Chinese medicine, hypertension is believed to result from energy blockages along the liver meridian.

Acupuncture is designed to free energy blockages by the insertion of needles into specific points on meridians known as acupoints. An acupoint is a point on a meridian where qi is concentrated and where qi can enter or leave the body.

HOW EFFECTIVE IS ACUPUNCTURE?
Research suggests that acupuncture can relieve stress by triggering the release of natural, heroinlike chemicals in the brain, and it can lower

blood pressure by having an effect on hormone secretion in the body. In a trial published in 1997, 50 people with untreated essential hypertension received acupuncture and, within 30 minutes, their blood pressure fell from an average of 169/107 mmHg to 151/96 mmHg (with a heart rate reduction from 77 to 72 beats per minute). Blood levels of renin (see page 16), a hormone involved in blood pressure regulation, also fell significantly.

Other studies have shown that acupuncture can improve the function of the left side of the heart, and that it's effective in some people for whom anti-hypertensive drugs have failed. Researchers in California have also shown acupuncture can blunt the increase in blood pressure caused by mental stress—in those receiving acupuncture, blood pressure rose by only 2.9 mmHg during periods of stress, as opposed to 5.4 mmHg in those receiving sham acupuncture.

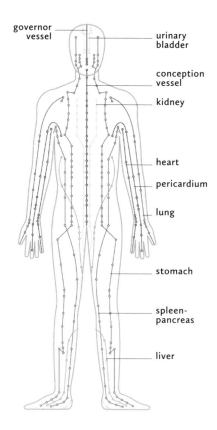

THE MERIDIANS
There are 12 pairs of meridians in the body. Acupuncture works by stimulating or suppressing the flow of qi energy along these channels at specific places known as acupoints. Blockages in the liver meridian are linked with hypertension.

governor vessel

urinary bladder

conception vessel

kidney

heart

pericardium

lung

stomach

spleen-pancreas

liver

CONSULTING AN ACUPUNCTURIST

During an initial consultation an acupuncturist will ask detailed questions about your health, emotional state, and your past health and family history. He or she will also assess the flow of qi through your meridians by taking your pulse (there are 12 wrist pulses, six on each wrist, as opposed to the single pulse used in Western medicine) and examining the general appearance, color, and texture of your tongue.

During acupuncture, a therapist stimulates (or sometimes suppresses) the flow of qi by inserting fine, sterile, disposable needles a fraction of an inch into your skin at selected acupoints. Although you might notice a slight pricking or tingling sensation as a needle is inserted, you should not feel any pain. Needles can be inserted for a few seconds, a few minutes, or up to an hour. They might be flicked or rotated to stimulate qi and

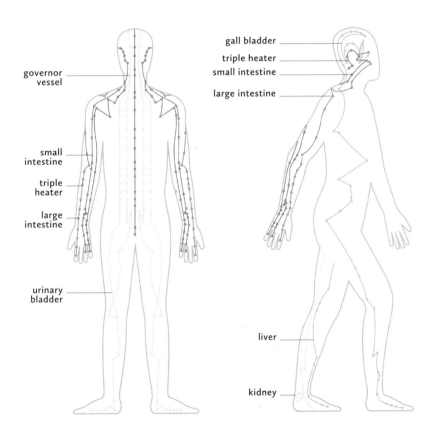

draw or disperse energy from an acupoint. In some cases, the action of the needles is enhanced with electricity (called electroacupuncture) or with a burning herb (called moxibustion). For a long-standing problem, such as hypertension, you will benefit from one or two treatments per week for at least two months.

ACUPRESSURE

You can stimulate acupoints yourself using finger or thumb pressure. This is known as acupressure and relies on the same underlying principles as acupuncture. Many people are more comfortable with acupressure than with the insertion of needles. You should avoid using acupressure if your blood pressure is 200/100 mmHg or higher. However, if your blood pressure is below this, try stimulating suitable acupoints—I suggest one in the box below and two more in the full-strength program on page 220.

ACUPRESSURE SELF-HELP
There is an acupoint in Chinese medicine known as LV3 or tai chong ("great surge") that lies on your liver meridian. Stimulating this point helps lower blood pressure by releasing stagnant energy along the liver meridian. To find LV3, place your index finger on the top of your foot, on the web of skin between your big toe and second toe. Then slide your finger ¾ inch along the top of your foot, until you feel a depression between the two underlying bones. Press on this point with your index finger.

YOGA

Yoga is an ancient Hindu system of philosophy that uses postures, breath control, and meditation to calm the mind and body. Although there are many different types of yoga, all have the ultimate aim of union between your inner self and the divine.

According to yogic theory, the practice of yoga enhances the flow of life-force energy around the body. This energy is known as prana and it flows along channels called nadis (in the same way that qi energy flows through meridians according to the Chinese view of the body; see page 55). When prana flows freely, the body exists in a state of health and balance; when prana is blocked, the body becomes ill.

One of the aims of yoga is to encourage prana to flow up a central channel, or nadi, in the body called sushumna nadi. This channel starts at the base of the body (the perineum) and ends at the crown of the head. Along this channel lie energy centers known as chakras—as energy ascends through each chakra, you experience a different state of consciousness. When energy reaches the crown chakra, you are said to have reached a higher level of consciousness in which you have moved beyond the self—this is the ultimate aim of all yoga.

From a Western perspective it's recognized that yoga is a powerful technique for reducing both stress and blood pressure. Yoga can also improve other risk factors for cardiovascular disease. A study published in 2005 showed that lifestyle interventions based on a variety of yoga asanas (postures), pranayama (breathing exercises), and relaxation techniques could produce significant improvements in blood glucose control and cholesterol levels within just nine days.

STARTING YOGA

Yoga is widely taught in the West. You can find classes in most health and leisure centers, as well as in dedicated yoga centers and retreats. For optimum benefit, yoga should be practiced three or four times a week for 30 to 60 minutes per session. Start slowly, however, in a beginner's class, and gradually increase the amount of time you practice. You can also teach yourself yoga at home. I include some simple yoga poses in Part Three that are beneficial for hypertension.

YOGA POSTURES TO AVOID
If your hypertension is not fully controlled, avoid inverted postures, such as headstands or shoulderstands. Inversion can temporarily increase blood pressure.

TYPES OF YOGA

When looking for a class, there are various types of yoga to choose from—some are more strenuous than others. Choose the type that best matches your fitness level.

HATHA YOGA

This concentrates on the performance of classical yoga postures and is the most widely practiced form of yoga in the West. In a typical class you will be taught poses that flow comfortably from one to another at your own pace. Classes are taught at different levels from beginners to advanced.

IYENGAR YOGA

This is a form of hatha yoga. It uses classical yoga postures with the emphasis on alignment and symmetry within individual postures. In an Iyengar class you will be taught how to use props, such as blocks, to help you get into postures correctly. This form of yoga is ideal for beginners, especially if you are not very fit. I recommend it if you're following the gentle or moderate program (see Part Three).

VINIYOGA

This is a slow, gentle form of yoga that does not stress your joints. Postures, breath awareness, movements, relaxation, meditation, and guided imagery are all used and are tailored to your individual needs. Viniyoga is ideal if you are unfit, middle-age or older, or stressed or recovering from illness. I recommend it if you're following the gentle program.

KRIPALU YOGA

This uses meditation and postural alignments to produce a continuous series of spontaneous, dynamic movements. Kripalu yoga is also gentle and relaxing, making it ideal for someone following the gentle or moderate program.

KUNDALINI YOGA

This form of yoga uses postures and breathing exercises along with

THE CHAKRAS

Chakras are energy centers that are situated along the midline of your body, from your perineum to the crown of your head. Practicing yoga encourages energy to move up through the chakras, bringing physical, emotional, and spiritual well-being. Each chakra is associated with particular benefits. For example, meditating on the root chakra, muladhara, releases physical and emotional tension.

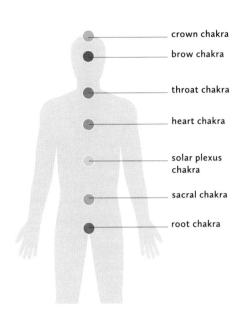

crown chakra

brow chakra

throat chakra

heart chakra

solar plexus chakra

sacral chakra

root chakra

mantras, meditation, visualization, and guided relaxation. It's ideal for those following the moderate program.

SIVANANDA YOGA

This uses a series of 12 different poses, relaxation techniques, mantras, and breathing exercises. It's ideal for someone flexible who is following the moderate or full-strength program.

ASHTANGA YOGA

This focuses on building strength, suppleness, and stamina and is also known as power yoga. You perform a sequence of postures that flow seamlessly one into another. Even beginners' classes in ashtanga yoga can be fairly strenuous, so this form of yoga is ideal if you're physically fit and following the full-strength program.

BIKRAM YOGA

This uses a sequence of yoga postures that are performed in a room heated to at least 100°F. It's designed to make you sweat profusely and should be avoided by people with hypertension.

QIGONG

Qigong, pronounced "chee gong," is often referred to as Chinese yoga. It has been practiced in China for more than 2,000 years. Qigong is based on the same principle that underlies other Chinese systems of healing, such as acupuncture: that life-force energy known as chi (or qi) flows through channels in the body called meridians. When qi flows smoothly we exist in a state of health and equilibrium, but when its flow is impeded, we become ill. The gentle movements that are characteristic of qigong are designed to regulate the flow of qi through the meridians. "Qi" translates as "energy" and "gong" means "work" or "cultivation."

Research shows that qigong can lower blood pressure (typically by 11/7 mmHg) and cholesterol levels, which makes it at least as effective as normal exercise. For people taking anti-hypertensive medication, practicing qigong has been shown to reduce the drug dosage required for blood pressure maintenance, as well as reducing the incidence of stroke.

STARTING QIGONG

Qigong is usually taught in tai chi classes (qigong movements are often used to warm up before practicing the flowing sequence of tai chi movements), but you can also learn qigong from a teacher who teaches

THE TAN TIEN

The tan tien is very important in qigong. It's the place inside the body where qi is stored—it's sometimes referred to as the energy powerhouse or reservoir—and it lies (1¼ inches) underneath your navel and about one third of the way inside your body in line with the top of your head. At the end of any qigong practice it's important to direct qi back into the tan tien—you do this using your hands, and also by visualizing the flow of qi back into this area. When the tan tien is full of qi, it pumps it in a circuit around the body bringing nourishment and well-being. If you go to classes to learn qigong, you will be taught to breathe deeply into your tan tien. Instead of breathing into your chest cavity, you will be encouraged to draw your breath deep down into your abdomen so your belly expands outward. Over time, this should become your default method of breathing.

privately. In the moderate program in Part Three, I provide a series of qigong exercises that are easy to do at home. Even if you don't do the moderate program, you can try the qigong exercises as a taster.

ASPECTS OF QIGONG

There are many different styles of qigong. Some styles concentrate on static standing postures, others on slow, fluid movements that are similar in appearance to tai chi. Still other styles emphasize meditation. But common to all styles of qigong is the importance that is placed on breathwork and mental focus or visualization. These are considered very important in regulating the flow of qi.

BREATHWORK

When you practise qigong, your breathing should be slow and deep, and penetrate as far as your tan tien (see box opposite). Allow your movements to fall in time with your breath, rather than the other way around.

MENTAL FOCUS

Visualizing the flow of qi in your body as you practise qigong can greatly enhance the benefits. When you become experienced in qigong, as well as visualizing qi you should be able to feel it flowing in your body—it might manifest itself as a tingling or warm sensation.

MEDITATION

Meditation is a practice that involves focusing the mind to achieve a state of calm and heightened awareness. Those experienced in meditation can quickly enter a trancelike state in which the brain generates special theta waves that are associated with creativity, visions, and profound relaxation. Meditation can be practiced by itself, but it often goes hand in hand with yoga in helping reduce blood pressure and the adverse effects of stress. At least 20 studies have shown meditation helps lower blood pressure in people with mild or moderate hypertension.

STARTING MEDITATION

You can learn meditation from a teacher or by yourself. I provide some simple meditation exercises that are suitable for everyone in Part Three. Ideally, you should try to meditate for 15 to 30 minutes for at least five days a week, and preferably every day.

TYPES OF MEDITATION

There are many different ways to meditate and many different traditions, both spiritual and secular, that teach meditation.

MINDFULNESS MEDITATION

This encourages you to focus on your breath to improve awareness of the present moment. You can also practice mindfulness in daily life by focusing on sensations, textures, colors, smells, and sounds around you.

MOVING MEDITATION

This involves quieting your mind through movement, such as walking. Movement engages your body and quiets your mind.

TRANSCENDENTAL MEDITATION (TM)

This was developed by Maharishi Mahesh Yogi to meet the needs of busy, modern lifestyles—TM is practiced twice a day, for 20 minutes each time. It uses the silent repetition of Sanskrit mantras to help you achieve a state of restful alertness. In 2005, a study showed that those practicing TM were 23 percent less likely to die from any cause, and 30 percent less likely to die from heart attack or stroke over an eight-year followup period, compared with a similar group of people not practicing TM.

RELAXATION RESPONSE MEDITATION

This was derived from TM by Dr Herbert Benson, a Harvard University researcher, who wanted to make this form of relaxation more acceptable to Westerners. He took the principles of TM and moved them out of an Eastern context. Instead of Sanskrit mantras, you choose words, such as "relax" or "peace," that are rooted in your own belief system.

BIOFEEDBACK AND AUTOGENIC TRAINING

Both biofeedback and autogenic training are therapies that, like meditation, help you lower your blood pressure using the power of your mind. During biofeedback, a practitioner will attach you to devices that monitor your body for sweat production, muscle tension and heart rate (this tells you how stressed or relaxed you are). Information from these devices is constantly fed back to you so you can monitor your level of stress/relaxation as you practice breathing techniques and relaxation exercises. If a particular relaxation exercise works for you, you'll immediately witness a drop in your muscle tension, and heart rate. Such feedback provides a direct and powerful way of learning how to relax. Most people learn to lower their blood pressure after just four to six biofeedback sessions.

Autogenic training works on a similar principle to biofeedback, but without the monitoring devices. See page 217 for an example of an autogenic training exercise.

NUTRITIONAL APPROACHES TO TREATMENT

A healthy diet can protect against hypertension and other cardiovascular problems by providing vitamins, minerals, antioxidants, and other substances (such as phytochemicals) that have a beneficial effect on body function. It's important to avoid eating too much of the wrong sort of food because this can damage your cardiovascular health in the following ways:

- If you're genetically predisposed to hypertension, excess salt can contribute to its development.
- Eating insufficient amounts of fiber increases the absorption of dietary cholesterol and can cause blood cholesterol levels to rise—this can lead to atherosclerosis.
- Eating too much food that contains hydrogenated fat and trans fats (see page 73) increases the risk of atherosclerosis.

- Eating too much carbohydrate raises triglyceride levels and stimulates the secretion of insulin, the main fat-storing hormone in the body. This can lead to weight gain and obesity—a risk factor for atherosclerosis.
- An insufficient amount of antioxidants in your diet contributes to the development of atherosclerosis.
- Insufficient amounts of folate and vitamins B6 and B12 are associated with elevated levels of homocysteine (see page 29), which, once again, promote the development of atherosclerosis.

EATING HEALTHILY

The guidelines for eating healthily when you have hypertension are based on the results of a series of studies called the Dietary Approaches to Stop Hypertension (DASH) trials. The emphasis in the "DASH diet" is on fruit, vegetables, whole grains, poultry, fish, and low-fat dairy products. The DASH diet recommends cutting down on red meat, saturated fat, cholesterol-rich foods, sodium, and sugar. If you follow this diet, you might see significant reductions in blood pressure in just eight weeks. Following the DASH diet not only lowers your blood pressure, it can also increase your levels of "good" cholesterol, lower triglyceride levels, and help you lose a significant amount of weight. The following guidelines encompass the principles of the DASH diet. I recommend you follow them every day.

EAT RAW OR LIVING FOODS

Where appropriate, make sure half the foods you eat are raw. Processing and cooking destroys antioxidants, vitamins, minerals, enzymes, and other phytochemicals, making foods less nutritious. Eat uncooked and unprocessed fruit, vegetables, salad, nuts, and seeds. Living foods such as sprouted beans and seeds (for example, alfalfa, radish, mung bean, broccoli, white radish, red-clover, wheat, lentil, quinoa, mustard, and cress) are high in enzyme and nutrient content because they are still growing. You can find out how to sprout your own beans and seeds on pages 154–155. If you eat raw fish (such as sushi or sashimi) or raw meat (such as steak tartare or carpaccio), make sure it's extremely fresh.

CONCENTRATE ON EATING FRUIT AND VEGETABLES

Aim to eat four to five servings *each* of fruit and vegetables per day. Fruit is an exceptionally good source of potassium, antioxidants, fiber, and phytochemicals, and has a blood pressure-lowering effect. Apples, avocados, blueberries, cherries, figs, grapefruit, grapes, guava, kiwi, mango, and pomegranate (see pages 81–85) are particularly recommended for people with hypertension. Similarly, certain vegetables (broccoli, mushrooms, and spinach) and legumes (chickpeas and soybeans) provide benefits for the circulatory system. Salad leaves that are red or dark green provide the most nutrients.

AVOID OVERCOOKING VEGETABLES

Any form of cooking destroys antioxidants, vitamins, and phytochemicals. Boiling, microwaving, or frying reduces the carotenoid/vitamin A content of food by 40 percent after one hour and by 70 percent after two hours (in casseroles, for example). Around 20 percent of folate in vegetables is lost during pressure-cooking and up to 50 percent during boiling and microwaving. Vitamin B2 in vegetables is readily lost into cooking water (it colors the water yellow), and when frozen vegetables are thawed and cooked, 40 percent of vitamin B6 is lost into water. Vitamin C is the most unstable nutrient—up to 50 percent is lost in cooking water when you boil vegetables. Light steaming or brief stir-frying is the best way to preserve nutrients. If you need to boil vegetables, add them to a small amount of boiling water, and cook briefly. Chopping them into coarse chunks rather than thin julienne strips also reduces the surface area over which nutrients are lost. You can reclaim lost nutrients by using cooking water in gravy, sauces, and stocks.

EAT HEALTHY FATS

Eat foods that are rich in omega-3 fatty acids (see page 74), such as oily fish and certain nuts and seeds. Nuts and seeds are rich not only in healthy fats but also in magnesium. A handful a day can reduce your risk of a heart attack or stroke. Almonds, Brazil nuts, pumpkin seeds, and walnuts (see pages 81–86) and their oils are particularly beneficial.

EAT ORGANIC WHEN YOU CAN

Ounce for ounce, organic foods consistently provide more nutrients—partly because they tend to contain less water, and partly because they are grown in soils fertilized with natural material rich in trace elements, rather than just the potassium, nitrogen, and phosphates in artificial fertilizer. Organic foods are also grown for flavor rather than uniformity of size, shape, and color.

CUT BACK ON SALT

This is one of the most important steps for your cardiovascular health. See my advice on salt intake on pages 76–77.

SELECT LOW-GLYCEMIC FOODS

These foods cause a slow and steady rise in your blood glucose level (as opposed to high-glycemic foods, which cause a sharp peak; see pages 77–80). Examples of low-glycemic foods include legumes, wholegrains, and brown rice. High-glycemic foods, which should be limited, include sugar, sweet or starchy foods, and potato products—they increase triglyceride levels and can lead to weight gain which is bad for your cardiovascular health.

SELECT SUPERFOODS

As well as fruit, vegetables, nuts, and seeds, certain other foods are beneficial for people with hypertension. These include dark chocolate, garlic (and related foods, especially shallots), green tea, oily fish, and yogurt with live cultures (see pages 80–86).

AVOID ADDITIVES

Whenever possible, avoid foods full of additives, such as artificial colorings, flavorings (especially monosodium glutamate), sweeteners (such as aspartame), and preservatives.

DRINK PLENTY OF FLUID

Aim to drink two to three quarts of fluid per day. Concentrate on drinking water, green tea, and unsweetened herbal or fruit teas. Cut back on caffeinated drinks, including coffee, and avoid carbonated drinks (other than water) as these often contain excessive amounts of phosphoric acid, glucose, and/or artificial sweeteners, colorings, and preservatives.

TAKE APPROPRIATE SUPPLEMENTS

Although the primary source of nutrients in your diet should be food, nutritional supplements can have a powerful protective effect on your circulatory health (see pages 86–92).

EATING MORE FRUIT AND VEGETABLES

Fruit and vegetables are excellent sources of vitamins, minerals, antioxidants, fiber, and plant substances (phytonutrients), all of which have beneficial effects on the circulation. A number of studies show that people with the highest intake of fruit and vegetables have the lowest blood pressure and the lowest risk of developing hypertension, coronary heart disease, and stroke.

One study involving 41,541 women with an initially normal blood pressure found that, over a four-year follow-up period, the more fruit and vegetables they ate, the lower their systolic and diastolic blood pressures, regardless of their weight, alcohol, and sodium intakes. Apples, oranges, prunes, grapes, carrots, alfalfa, mushrooms, raw spinach, tofu, and celery were the fruit and vegetables associated with the most significant reductions in blood pressure.

THE POWER OF ANTIOXIDANTS

During normal bodily processes the body produces substances known as free radicals. In excess, free radicals can cause damage to cells throughout the body and lead to the hardening and furring up of the arteries (excess free-radical production can be the result of stress, illness, and exposure to tobacco smoke and pollution, among other things). However, the antioxidants present in fruit and vegetables can neutralize free radicals and prevent the damage they would otherwise do to the body. An antioxidant-rich diet is very important for the health of the heart and blood vessels—a number of studies show that people with hypertension are likely to have low levels of antioxidants.

The main antioxidants in fruit and vegetables are vitamins C and E, beta-carotene (which is converted to the antioxidant vitamin A in the body), and the mineral selenium. But there are also many other equally important antioxidants found in plants. Examples include:

- Polyphenols—found in red grapes, blueberries,and cranberries.
- Proanthocyanidins—found in berries and grapes.
- Lycopene—found in tomatoes.
- Quercetin—found in apples, onions, and citrus fruit.
- Lutein—found in green leafy vegetables, such as spinach and kale.

OTHER PROTECTIVE EFFECTS

A high intake of fruit and vegetables can protect your cardiovascular system by providing you with an excellent source of the mineral potassium. Your kidneys need potassium to flush excess sodium from your body—this is important because excess sodium is strongly linked to age-related rises in blood pressure.

Fruit and vegetables also provide folate, a B-group vitamin. This is the natural form of synthetic folic acid, and it's vital for regulating blood levels of a substance called homocysteine (high levels of homocysteine are linked with cardiovascular disease; see page 29).

In addition, plant hormones called phytoestrogens have a weak, estrogenlike action on hormone receptors in the circulation. They have been shown to dilate coronary arteries, enhance heart function, reduce blood levels of harmful LDL-cholesterol (see pages 72–73), and reduce blood stickiness. They also possess antioxidant and anti-inflammatory properties. Research consistently shows an association between phytoestrogen-rich diets and a reduced risk of cardiovascular disease.

A high fruit and vegetable intake insures you get plenty of plant fiber. This helps slow the absorption of dietary carbohydrates and fats, so the level of glucose and fats in your blood remains stable. This, in turn, reduces your risk of atherosclerosis (see pages 19–20), and, therefore, hypertension. Plant fiber also encourages a beneficial balance of intestinal bacteria needed to convert phytoestrogens to more powerful forms.

EATING ENOUGH FRUIT AND VEGETABLES

The Dietary Guidelines for Americans recommends the quantities of food that should be eaten daily as part of a healthy diet. These quantities vary according to gender, age, and level of physical activity. Specific recommendations are given in the Department of Agriculture's Food Pyramid. You can view the details and print copies of the pyramid at www.mypyramid.gov. You can also try the following suggestions:

- Add fruit, such as bananas and grapes, to your breakfast cereal, or stir raspberries into yogurt.
- Make salad the basis of your lunch.
- Include several different types of vegetable in your evening meal. Experiment with vegetables you might not have tried before, such as bok choy.
- Whenever possible, replace red meat with vegetables—vegetarians and lactovegetarians have lower blood pressure than the general population, regardless of their age, gender, and weight.
- Snack on fruit or vegetables (tomatoes, cucumbers, or slices of red pepper) when you feel hungry.

WHAT COUNTS AS A SERVING?

Over a period of time, build up to eating the optimum number of cups of fruit and vegetables a day, as listed in the Food Pyramid. Try to make your selection as varied as possible, rather than eating, say, just apples or bananas each day. The following amounts give you an idea of how much fruit or vegetables constitute "a serving." However, another interpretation of a serving is that it's the amount you are happy to eat in one sitting. Generally, the bigger the fruit or vegetable serving, the better. Potatoes do not count toward a vegetable serving as they consist mainly of starch.

The same is true of yams. Legumes are counted as a vegetable serving but, unless they are sprouted, they contain little vitamin C. Here are examples of a 1-cup serving:

- Generally, a 1-cup serving of fruit equals 1 cup chopped fresh fruit; ½ cup dried fruit; or 1 cup 100% fruit juice.
- ½ large or 1 small apple.
- 1 large banana; 1 large peach; 2 large or 3 medium plums; 1 medium pear.
- 32 seedless grapes; 8 large strawberries.
- Generally a 1-cup serving of vegetables equals 1 cup cooked or raw chopped vegetables; 1 cup vegetable juice; 2 cups leafy greens.
- 3 spears broccoli.
- 2 medium carrots.
- 1 large baked potato or sweet potato.
- 8 ounces tofu.
- 1 large ear corn.
- 1 large red or green bell pepper.

EATING GOOD FATS

How much fat—and what type—you eat in your daily diet can have a big impact on your long-term health. Some types of fat cause blood levels of unhealthy cholesterol to rise and can lead to clogged and narrowed arteries (or damage them further if you have atherosclerosis). Other types of fat can actually improve the health of your cardiovascular system and reduce your future risk of coronary heart disease.

UNHEALTHY FATS
When hypertension is diagnosed a blood test is carried out to check the levels of certain types of fat in the blood: triglycerides, LDL-cholesterol, and HDL-cholesterol (see the box opposite and the chart on page 74 for recommended levels of each). Unhealthy levels of these fats exacerbate

GOOD VERSUS BAD CHOLESTEROL

Good cholesterol is known as HDL-cholesterol (high-density lipoprotein). It's considered good because it transports excess bad cholesterol back to the liver where it can be disposed of. Bad cholesterol is known as LDL-cholesterol (low-density lipoprotein). When it reaches a certain level in your blood, it can start to deposit itself on the inner artery walls, which, over time, blocks your arteries. The ratio of your LDL and HDL levels is important in health terms—if you have high LDL/low HDL, your risk of coronary heart disease increases. You can change this by eating healthily, cutting down on alcohol, exercising, and not smoking.

hypertension and increase the risk of developing cardiovascular problems. Although your family history, and other factors, can affect whether you develop unhealthy levels of blood fats, your diet plays an important part (and one that is within your control). The following types of dietary fat can increase your risk:

SATURATED FATS

These are fats that tend to be solid at room temperature. They are found in cheese, butter, lard, meat, eggs, and palm oil, as well as being present in many processed foods, such as cakes, cookies, pies, and pastries. A diet that is high in saturated fat can lead to weight gain and, in some cases, is linked with an increase in the bad type of cholesterol (LDL-cholesterol).

TRANS FATS

These are formed when polyunsaturated oils are partly solidified to make vegetable shortening or margarine in a process called hydrogenation. Trans fats have a molecular structure that hastens the hardening and furring up of the arteries, raises blood levels of bad LDL-cholesterol, and lowers levels of good HDL-cholesterol. Trans fats are linked with an increased risk of hypertension and coronary heart disease. The USDA has determined there is no safe level of trans fats in a healthy diet, and now requires trans-fat levels to be included in nutritional labeling.

HEALTHY FATS

Replacing saturated and trans fats with healthy fats can have a positive impact on your blood fat levels and reduce your chance of health problems.

POLYUNSATURATED FATS

These are fats that are liquid at room temperature. They include vegetable oils, such as corn and sunflower oils. They contain essential fatty acids such as omega-6 and omega-3 fatty acids, both of which are important in the prevention and control of a range of diseases from arthritis to heart disease and cancer. Some polyunsaturated fats lower the levels of bad LDL-cholesterol in your blood. However, too many omega-6 fatty acids in your diet can have the opposite effect and cause damage to your body. For this reason, it's advisable to prioritize monounsaturated fats and omega-3s over omega-6 polyunsaturated fats.

OMEGA-3 FATTY ACIDS

These are found in polyunsaturated fats, but they deserve special mention because they play such an important role in protecting your heart. Omega-3s are found in walnuts, flaxseeds, and flaxseed oil, and in oily fish such as mackerel, herring, tuna, salmon, and trout. Because omega-3s are so important for cardiovascular health, I advise anyone with hypertension to take a fish oil supplement (see my supplement advice in each of the three programs in Part Three).

HEALTHY LEVELS OF FATS IN YOUR BLOOD

Type of fat	Recommended level
Total cholesterol	Below 200 mg/dl
Triglycerides	Below 150 mg/dl
LDL-cholesterol	Below 100 mg/dl
HDL-cholesterol	Above 60 mg/dl

HEALTHY NUT BUTTERS

Everyone is familiar with peanut butter, but did you know that whole food stores and online stores sell other butters, too? These include almond, Brazil nut, macadamia, hazelnut, pistachio, and even pumpkin seed butters. Some, especially walnut butter, need refrigeration before you open them to preserve their nutritional qualities. They are a rich source of monounsaturated fats, protein, and antioxidants—especially vitamin E. Buy nut butters that are free from salt, sugar, and preservatives, and are preferably organic. For a simple lunch, spread nut butter on a few crackers and serve with a light salad and fruit.

MONOUNSATURATED FATS

These are liquid at room temperature, but can solidify at lower temperatures (in the refrigerator, for example). They include olive oil, canola oil, and peanut oil. Monounsaturated fats are also found in olives, avocados, and some nuts (especially macadamias) and seeds. They not only lower your level of bad LDL-cholesterol; they also maintain or even raise the level of good HDL-cholesterol in your blood.

FATS IN YOUR DAY-TO-DAY DIET

If you are accustomed to a diet that is high in saturated fat, the eating plans I suggest later on in the book (see Part Three) will ease you into a lower-fat way of eating, with the emphasis on monounsaturated fats, such as olive oil, avocados, nuts, and seeds. When you go shopping, get into the habit of checking food labels for the fat content of foods (do the same for salt and sugar). The amount of fat you eat each day depends on your age, gender, and the amount of physical activities you do. Don't forget the total amount of fat you consume includes that "hidden" in prepared foods, not just what you cook with or spread on bread.

- Each food label will give a percentage of the Daily Value (DV) of different nutrients in that food, based on a 2,000 calorie diet.
- The % DV for total fat includes all kinds of fat.
- 20% DV for total fat, or greater, is high.
- 5% DV for total fat, or less, is low.

CUTTING DOWN ON SALT

We need salt (sodium chloride) for nerve and muscle activity and to maintain the water balance in the body. The problem is that many of us consume too much of it. Today, salt consumption in people following a Western diet is can be as high as 12 grams per day. Yet, we evolved on a diet that provided less than 1 gram of salt a day, and an average adult weighing 154 pounds can maintain a healthy sodium balance with an intake of as little as 1.25 grams of salt per day—as long as he or she does not sweat heavily.

A high salt consumption is a major cause of the age-related rise in blood pressure that is common in the West. Populations with salt intakes of less than 3 grams per day do not have this age-related rise.

HOW SALT CAUSES DAMAGE

A high-salt diet causes fluid retention, which, in turn, raises blood pressure. And, in genetically sensitive individuals, consuming too much salt can cause the arteries to stiffen and narrow, and the left ventricle of the heart to thicken so the heart has to work harder to pump blood. These changes contribute to and exacerbate hypertension.

Researchers estimate that reducing salt intake by $\frac{1}{10}$ ounce per day can reduce the incidence of stroke by 13 percent and of coronary heart disease by 10 percent. Reducing salt intake by $\frac{1}{5}$ ounce per day can double this benefit, and reducing salt intake by $\frac{3}{10}$ ounce per day could potentially triple this benefit.

HOW TO CUT DOWN

Avoid adding table salt to food during cooking, and never put a salt shaker on the dining table. Researchers have found if you stop doing this, blood pressure is reduced by at least 5 mmHg. Just this simple step can reduce the incidence of coronary heart disease by 15 percent, and the incidence of stroke by 26 percent within the general population.

Also avoid obviously salty foods, such as potato chips, bacon, or salted nuts; fish or meats cured with salt; and products canned in brine.

CHECK FOOD LABELS FOR SALT CONTENT

Most Americans consume between 4,000 to 6,000 mg sodium per day, and the maximum recommended is 2,400, or slightly more than one teaspoon, although it should be even less if you suffer from high blood pressure. Processed foods are particularly high in their sodium content, so it pays to carefully read labels. "Sodium free or no sodium" means each serving has less than 5 mg sodium and no sodium chloride in the ingredients; "very low sodium" means 35 mg or less per serving; "low sodium" is 140 mg or less per serving; "reduced sodium" or "less sodium" means each serving contains 25 percent less sodium than a regular product.

Even meat bouillon, pâtés, cubes, and yeast extracts have a high salt content and are best avoided.

ADAPTING TO LESS SALT

Experiments show that if you're accustomed to highly salted foods, it takes at least one month for salt receptors on your tongue to readjust and start detecting lower salt concentrations. As a result, foods can taste bland during this time. Don't be tempted to add salt—use freshly ground black pepper, garlic, and herbs and spices to add flavor instead. Soon you will start to become more sensitive to the natural flavor in your food. Adding lime juice to food can also help by decreasing the concentration at which your taste buds can detect salt.

FOLLOWING A LOW-GLYCEMIC DIET

Foods vary in the effect they have on the level of glucose in your blood— some cause a slow, steady, sustained rise in blood glucose, while others cause fast peaks followed by troughs. Foods in the former category are referred to as "low glycemic," and it's now generally accepted that a low-glycemic diet is good for your long-term health. I also recommend a low-glycemic diet to anyone who wants to lose weight. In contrast, if you eat a lot of high-glycemic foods that make your blood glucose rise quickly, in the long term this can damage your blood vessels and promote the development of atherosclerosis.

How a food affects your blood glucose depends on how much carbohydrate it contains, and what type. "Complex" carbohydrates, such as brown rice, consist of chains of sugars that are broken down relatively slowly and cause a sustained rise in your blood glucose. "Simple" carbohydrates, found in cakes and confectionery, for example, are rapidly absorbed into your circulation and quickly raise your blood glucose level. Simple carbohydrates are also referred to as simple sugars, and these are the carbohydrate foods I recommend that you avoid or eat in moderation.

WHAT IS GLYCEMIC INDEX?

In 1981 scientists at the University of Toronto developed the glycemic index (GI) as a way of ranking foods to show how quickly or slowly they cause blood glucose to rise. They gave glucose a rating of 100 (glucose is the simplest type of sugar and is absorbed the most quickly). The researchers then compared how other foods affected blood glucose and rated them accordingly. For example, a food that raised blood glucose levels half as much as glucose was given a GI value of 50. Foods containing lots of simple sugars were given the highest GI rating: 70 or higher. Foods with a low GI, of less than 55, contain carbohydrates that break down more slowly and therefore have only a minor effect on blood glucose levels.

WHAT IS GLYCEMIC LOAD?

Although GI ratings give us guidance about the effects of different foods on blood glucose, critics point out that GI is not a perfect system. A good way of demonstrating the flaw in the GI system is to look at the example of carrots. They have a middle range GI of 47, yet they would be unlikely to cause a noticeable rise in blood glucose simply because people tend to eat so few of them in one sitting. You need to eat about two bunches of carrots to produce the blood glucose rise that would be expected from a GI of 47. As a result of the flaws in the GI system, researchers at Harvard University developed the concept of the "glycemic load" (GL), which

GLYCEMIC VALUES OF SOME COMMON FOODS

FOOD	GLYCEMIC INDEX VALUE	GLYCEMIC LOAD VALUE
parsnips	97	12
baked potatoes	85	26
wholewheat bread	71	9
fresh pineapple	59	7
wholewheat rye bread	58	8
oatmeal	58	13
fresh apricots	57	4.9
muesli	56	9
honey	55	10
brown rice	55	18
kiwi	53	6
bananas	52	12
unsweetened orange juice	52	12
mangoes	51	8
new potatoes, boiled	50	14
mixed-grain bread	49	6
peas	48	3
carrots	47	3
grapes	46	8
sweet potatoes	44	11
oranges	42	5
unsweetened apple juice	40	11
apples	38	6
pears	38	4
wholewheat spaghetti	37	16
dried apricots	31	9

takes into account the amount of food eaten in a typical serving. The glycemic load is calculated by multiplying a food's glycemic-index value by the amount of carbohydrate found in a typical serving, then dividing the result by 100.

Foods with a GL value of 20 or more are classed as high GL, foods with values of 11 to 19 are medium GL, and foods with a value of 10 or less are low GL. Using this system, carrots receive a value of three, which means they have a negligible effect on blood glucose and can, therefore, be eaten in abundance. Books providing GI and GL values are widely available. I have also included some values of common foods in the chart on the right.

YOUR DAILY DIET

Aim to avoid foods with a high GI/GL and, instead, choose those foods that have a moderate to low ranking. You can also combine foods with a high GI/GL, such as baked potatoes, with those that have a lower GI/GL, such as beans, fish, green vegetables, meat, or nuts. This helps prevent fast peaks in your blood glucose levels.

In general, It's a good idea to cut down on the amount of sugar you eat in your daily diet. Avoid convenience foods, and try not to add sugar to drinks, such as tea and coffee. Reduce the amount of sugar you use in home-cooked recipes. Be aware of the amount of sugar in convenience foods; not just soft drinks, cakes, and cookies, but also breakfast cereals and canned products, such as baked beans. When you go shopping get into the habit of checking the "Nutrition Facts" label on all the food you buy for sugar content.

SUPERFOODS FOR HYPERTENSION

The following foods are considered "superfoods," and I recommend that you include as many as possible in your daily diet. Each one contains valuable nutrients or phytochemicals that have a positive effect on high blood pressure or improve the health of your heart and blood vessels generally. The inclusion of chocolate and wine might surprise you, but evidence suggests both have a beneficial effect on your cardiovascular system, providing you don't consume too much, and providing you eat dark chocolate and drink red wine.

SUPERFOOD	CARDIOVASCULAR BENEFITS	HOW TO USE IT
Almonds Contain vitamin E and antioxidants.	A handful of almonds a day can lower LDL-cholesterol by 4–5 percent and increase HDL-cholesterol by 6 percent. Almond oil has similar benefits. Eating nuts frequently can decrease the risk of coronary heart disease by 30–50 percent.	Eat a handful a day as a snack (about 23 kernels). Or grind to a powder to add to shakes and smoothies, or to sprinkle over cereals and desserts. Use almond oil in salad dressings.
Apples One of the richest dietary sources of antioxidant flavonoids, such as quercetin. Despite a relatively high content of fruit sugar, apples have a low GI value, which helps to stabilize blood glucose levels.	Eating an apple a day can reduce the risk of death from any cause at any age (but especially from coronary heart disease or stroke) by one-third, compared with those eating less.	Snack on apples, dried apple rings or apple "chips". Grate apple flesh and add it to salads and coleslaw (mix it with lemon juice to prevent browning). Use apple in Bircher muesli (see page 142).
Avocados Contain monounsaturated fat, essential fatty acids and vitamin E. A rich source of potassium. Note: avocados can interact with MAO inhibitors (a type of antidepressant drug) to increase blood pressure.	Daily consumption can increase beneficial HDL-cholesterol by 11 percent within a week. Avocado also boosts your absorption of phytonutrients – if you eat avocado in combination with spinach, your absorption of antioxidant carotenoids is quadrupled.	Use an avocado slicer to remove flesh from the skin easily. Drizzle with walnut or olive oil and eat as a salad. Add avocado flesh to salads. Mix with berries for an interesting fruit salad. Mash to make dips or simply to spread on oatcakes.

SUPERFOOD	CARDIOVASCULAR BENEFITS	HOW TO USE IT
Blueberries Rich in antioxidants known as anthocyanins and proanthocyanidins.	Daily consumption of 2 cups significantly lowers LDL-cholesterol and blood pressure (by inhibiting the production of angiotensin-converting enzyme; see page 16).	Add a handful of berries to yogurt, muesli, fromage blanc, fruit salads or any other dessert. Make your own fresh blueberry juice or smoothie.
Brazil nuts The richest dietary source of antioxidant selenium—a single nut contains around 50mcg. Also a good source of magnesium.	Eating nuts frequently can decrease the risk of coronary heart disease by 30–50 percent.	Eat as a snack, or chop and add to cereal, yogurts, and salads. Buy little and often for maximum freshness. Brazil nut butter is a delicious spread.
Broccoli A rich source of folate, phytoestrogens, vitamin C, calcium and magnesium.	The high antioxidant content helps lower blood pressure.	Eat raw, in salads, or lightly steamed or stir-fried.
Cherries (black) Provide antioxidant anthocyanins. A good source of vitamin C, plus useful amounts of potassium.	Cherries are thought to have the same health benefits as blueberries.	Eat as a snack, or add to fruit salads and other desserts. Use the flesh when making mixed fruit juices and smoothies.
Chickpeas A rich source of antioxidant isoflavones.	Regular intake can reduce total cholesterol and LDL-cholesterol by 4 percent.	Add to soups, stews, and salads. Mash to make hummus (see page 195).
Chocolate (dark) A rich source of flavonoids—ounce for ounce, dark chocolate has five times more antioxidant activity than blueberries.	Research found that older men who drank the most cocoa had a blood pressure that was 3.7/2.1mmHg lower than those who drank the least cocoa. They were also half as likely to die of cardiovascular (or any other illness) during a 15-year follow-up.	Eat about 1 ounce of dark chocolate (at least 70 percent cocoa solids) daily. If you are trying to lose weight, make sure you count the calories in chocolate as part of your daily intake. Drinking unsweetened cocoa is beneficial, too.

SUPERFOOD	CARDIOVASCULAR BENEFITS	HOW TO USE IT
Coconut Rich in medium-chain fatty acids—these aid the absorption of calcium and magnesium, and are used by the liver as a fuel. Because they are not converted into fat, they increase energy levels and aid weight loss.	Drinking coconut water has been shown to reduce systolic blood pressure by 71 percent and diastolic blood pressure by 29 percent.	Select virgin coconut oil (not odorless, hydrogenated versions) for the greatest health benefits. Use instead of margarine, butter and other oils when cooking and baking. Some experts suggest an intake of approx. 2oz. daily.
Figs Rich in polyphenol antioxidants, calcium, potassium and fiber. Ounce for ounce, dried figs contain more calcium than milk.	Antioxidants prevent oxidation of LDL-cholesterol. The beneficial effect lasts for four hours after consumption.	Eat fresh or dried for an energy-rich snack.
Garlic Contains important active ingredients, such as allicin.	Allicin lowers cholesterol levels and blood pressure and makes arteries more elastic.	Eat two or three cloves a day. Add to dishes during cooking. Try the recipe for garlic chicken on page 145.
Grapefruit Rich in vitamin C and antioxidants (particularly red grapefruit). See caution on page 120.	One grapefruit a day (either flesh or juice) significantly lowers LDL cholesterol.	Eat as a starter; add to fruit salads; drink freshly squeezed juice.
Grapes (red or black) Contain antioxidant anthocyanins and phytochemicals, such as resveratrol, plus potassium and magnesium.	Resveratrol helps lower blood pressure and prevent hardening and furring of the arteries.	Eat a handful of grapes a day or drink a glass of red grape juice. Drinking a glass of red wine daily also provides health benefits.
Green or white tea Contains powerful flavonoid antioxidants such as catechins.	Lowers LDL-cholesterol, blood pressure and blood stickiness. Reduces the risk of heart attack and stroke.	Drink throughout the day. Use left-over cold tea to soak dried fruit, as a base for sauces, soups or stews, or to make ice cream.

SUPERFOOD	CARDIOVASCULAR BENEFITS	HOW TO USE IT
Guava An excellent source of antioxidant carotenoids, vitamin C, potassium, and soluble fiber. Pink guava has an exceptionally high antioxidant content.	Eating several a day for three months has been found to reduce LDL-cholesterol by 10 percent, triglycerides by 8 percent, and blood pressure by 9/8mmHg; and to raise HDL-cholesterol by 8 percent.	Eat for breakfast and add to fruit salads. Drink fresh guava juice or add to smoothies.
Kiwi Rich in vitamins C and E, antioxidant polyphenols, and potassium.	Eating 2 or 3 kiwis a day for 28 days has been found to reduce the potential for abnormal blood clotting by 18 percent, and to lower triglycerides by 15 percent.	Eat with the top cut off, like a boiled egg. Add to fruit and vegetable salads. Include in juices and smoothies.
Mango A rich source of antioxidant carotenoids, and vitamins C and E. Also a good source of potassium.	Reduces the constriction of smooth muscle cells in artery walls and can, therefore, reduce stress-related rises in blood pressure.	Eat fresh in fruit salads or on its own. Dried mango makes a deliciously healthy sweet snack.
Mushrooms A good source of potassium and selenium. Contain a form of fiber (chitin), plus beta-glutan, which boosts general immunity.	Chitin can lower LDL-cholesterol. Some edible mushrooms, such as *Tricholoma giganteum* (a common species in Japan and Australia), reishi, and maitake, can lower blood pressure by blocking angiotensin-converting enzyme (see page 16).	Slice raw into salads; sauté in olive oil with garlic; parboil in bouillon; or bake in the oven, stuffed with mashed butternut squash and parsley. Take reishi or maitake as supplements.
Oats A rich source of soluble fiber, beta-glucan, and B vitamins.	One bowl of oatmeal a day can reduce LDL-cholesterol by 8–23 percent and reduce blood pressure by 7.5/5.5mmHg over 6 weeks.	Eat oatmeal for breakfast; mix uncooked oatmeal into yogurt; make homemade unsweetened muesli.
Oily fish A rich source of the omega-3 fatty acids (EPA and DHA), plus vitamins A, D and E.	Eating fish once a week can reduce the risk of a heart attack and stroke.	Eat very fresh fish raw, broiled, or baked.

SUPERFOOD	CARDIOVASCULAR BENEFITS	HOW TO USE IT
Olive oil A rich source of monounsaturated fats such as oleic acid. Extra virgin olive oil, made from the first olive pressing, has the highest antioxidant content.	A diet rich in olive oil reduces the risk of coronary heart disease by 25 percent and the risk of a second heart attack by 56 percent.	Use plain olive oil for cooking. Use extra virgin olive oil in salad dressings and for drizzling on food, and for dipping with bread.
Pomegranate One of the richest dietary sources of polyphenols, anthocyanins and tannins. A good source of vitamins C and E, carotenoids, and iron.	Drinking a glass of pomegranate juice a day lowers LDL-cholesterol and can reverse hardening of the arteries. In people with hypertension, drinking 2 tbsp. pomegranate juice twice a day can reduce systolic blood pressure by 5 percent.	Look for fresh pomegranate juice drinks, or make your own. Add pomegranate berries to salads or snack on them.
Pumpkin seeds Rich in vitamin E, zinc, and a substance called beta-sitosterol.	Beta-sitosterol lowers cholesterol. Eating pumpkin seeds can improve the activity of two groups of anti-hypertensive drugs: calcium channel blockers and ACE inhibitors, producing beneficial therapeutic effects and slowing the progression of hypertension.	Eat a handful as a snack or sprinkle onto salads and cereals. Grind and add to shakes and smoothies.
Soybeans A rich source of phytoestrogens (isoflavones).	Evidence shows that consuming 1½oz. soybean protein a day can reduce blood pressure by 7.88/5.27 mmHg within 12 weeks in people with hypertension, and by 2.34/1.28 mmHg in those without hypertension.	Use soybeans in soups, stews and stir-fries; eat products rich in soybean protein, such as tofu and vegetarian meals (but check salt content first). Add soybean protein powder to smoothies.
Spinach One of the richest dietary sources of the carotenoid antioxidants lutein and zeaxanthin.	Substances that inhibit angiotensin-converting enzyme (ACE; see page 34) have been isolated from spinach.	Eat raw or lightly steamed as an accompaniment to any meal. Baby leaves are great in salads. Try to eat one portion of a dark green leafy vegetable every day.

SUPERFOOD	CARDIOVASCULAR BENEFITS	HOW TO USE IT
Walnuts Rich in omega-6 and omega-3 fatty acids.	Regular consumption lowers LDL-cholesterol enough to decrease the risk of coronary heart disease by 30–50 percent and increase life span by an estimated 5–10 years.	Add to breakfast cereals, yogurt, and salads. Eat as a snack. Use walnut oil as a salad dressing.
Wine (red) Rich in antioxidant pigments.	Prevents blood clotting and atherosclerosis; increases levels of HDL-cholesterol.	Drink a glass ($\frac{2}{3}$ cup) a day.
Yogurt Yogurt with live cultures provides probiotic bacteria, calcium, magnesium, and potassium.	Probiotic bacteria can reduce hypertension by blocking angiotensin-converting enzyme (ACE).	Add to cereals and desserts; stir into soups; use in dressings and smoothies. Eat one 6oz. container per day.

SUPPLEMENTS FOR HYPERTENSION

The following charts summarize what I think are the most important supplements for people with hypertension. I explain the role of each supplement, together with the research findings that support its efficacy. I also suggest daily doses. You will find these supplements in my gentle, moderate, and full-strength programs in Part Three—there I recommend different dosages for each program.

Many of the following supplements—like the superfoods on the previous pages—are beneficial because they have an antioxidant action in the body. Antioxidants preserve the health of your cardiovascular system and prevent premature aging.

Although a healthy diet should always be the main way to obtain nutrients, food alone often does not supply the quantities of antioxidants, vitamins, and minerals needed for optimum protection. Many of the foods we eat in a contemporary Western diet are refined and processed, meaning they have lost many of the vitamins and minerals they started out with.

Supplements are widely available in drug stores, supermarkets, and whole-food stores. They are best taken immediately after food (just four bites of food or a glass of juice will do). If you have not eaten for more than 20 minutes, don't take a supplement. Wait until you have a snack or drink some juice, and then take it. If taken on an empty stomach, some supplements can make you feel sick or cause indigestion. It's not advisable to take supplements with coffee or tea, as these may interfere with absorption. For tips on how to remember your supplements, see page 118.

When you are taking two or more capsules of the same preparation a day, spread these out over the day, to maximize absorption and obtain more even blood levels of the supplement.

Do not take supplements during pregnancy or breastfeeding, except under the advice of a medical herbalist or nutritional therapist. If taking any prescribed medications, check with a pharmacist for any potential supplement-drug interactions.

SUPPLEMENT	RESEARCH FINDINGS	DOSE AND COMMENT
Vitamin C An important antioxidant nutrient that combats damage caused by free radicals. A sufficient vitamin C intake also controls the level of the stress hormone cortisol in your bloodstream.	Blood levels of vitamin C have a strong association with systolic blood pressure. People with the lowest blood levels of vitamin C have the highest blood pressure. Research has demonstrated adding 2 g vitamin C daily to an anti-hypertensive drug regime can lower systolic blood pressure by 13 mmHg after one month (compared with people who were taking an inactive placebo). The mechanism by which vitamin C lowers blood pressure is not yet understood.	*500–2,000 mg daily* High doses of vitamin C can result in indigestion. You can avoid this by selecting a supplement described as "nonacidic ester-C." Taking vitamin C supplements can affect laboratory results during some urine or stool tests, so make sure you tell your doctor if you are taking vitamin C.

SUPPLEMENT	RESEARCH FINDINGS	DOSE AND COMMENT
Vitamin E An important antioxidant that protects body fats from undergoing damaging oxidation.	Among 2000 people who had previously had a heart attack, those who were given vitamin E supplements for 18 months had a 77 percent lower risk of an additional heart attack—in fact, their risk dropped to the level where it was no greater than for people without coronary heart disease. Taking 67 mg vitamin E daily for at least two years reduces the risk of coronary heart disease by 40 percent. Centenarians have exceptionally high blood levels of vitamin E, which might contribute to their longevity.	*100–600 mg daily* Vitamin E is temporarily converted into a free radical as a result of its antioxidant action. For this reason it's important to take it alongside other antioxidants, such as vitamin C, so it's converted back into its antioxidant form.
Carotenoids These are the yellow-orange-red pigments in plants. Examples of carotenoids include beta-carotene in carrots, lycopene in tomatoes, and lutein in spinach and kale. Carotenoids have an antioxidant action in the body.	A large, international study covering 10 European countries found a significant link between low levels of lycopene levels and increased risk of heart attack. Lycopene-rich tomato extracts can reduce blood pressure by 10/4 mmHg within 8 weeks.	Mixed carotenoids: *15 mg daily* Lycopene-rich carotenoids: *15 mg daily* An excess intake of carotenoids can cause yellowness of the skin, but this resolves when the dose is reduced.
Coenzyme Q10 Improves oxygen uptake and energy production in cells. Acts together with vitamin E. Coenzyme Q10 is essential if you are taking a statin drug (see page 35), as these switch off co enzyme Q10 production.	Taking 100mg daily can reduce blood pressure by an average of 10.6/7.7 mmHg. One study showed that half of people with hypertension taking 225 mg coenzyme Q10 daily achieved a reduction of at least 1 (and up to 3) anti-hypertensive drugs within four and a half months.	*10–120 mg (or more) daily* In some trials people have taken 600 mg coenzyme Q10 daily with no adverse effects. Alpha lipoic acid, L-carnitine and coenzyme Q10 work synergistically and are often taken together.

SUPPLEMENT	RESEARCH FINDINGS	DOSE AND COMMENT
Selenium A mineral essential for the function of five major antioxidant enzymes in the body (known as glutathione peroxidases).	Selenium reduces blood clotting, which protects against coronary heart disease and stroke. Selenium levels are 27 percent lower in people with hypertension and 30 percent lower in those with coronary heart disease compared with healthy individuals. A five-year study of 1,110 Finnish males (55–74 years) found that a low selenium level almost quadrupled the risk of fatal stroke.	*50–200 mcg daily* Avoid taking more than the recommended dose of selenium. Excess is toxic.
Alpha lipoic acid Also known as thioctic acid, this is a powerful antioxidant that is involved in energy production in cells. It regenerates other important antioxidants such as vitamins C and E.	Alpha lipoic acid helps lower blood pressure by reducing the effect of excess sodium on the body (see page 76). Several studies suggest that alpha lipoic acid can reduce oxidative stress and the loss of protein in urine (which may be a sign that hypertension has damaged kidney function). It may therefore protect the kidneys in people with hypertension.	*100–600 mg daily* Alpha lipoic acid is often combined with l-carnitine (see page 90) in a 1:1 ratio. If you have diabetes, monitor your blood glucose level when you take alpha lipoic acid, as it stimulates the uptake of glucose into your muscle cells to lower blood glucose levels.
Magnesium A vital mineral for maintaining the correct salt balance and electrical stability across cell membranes. It is involved in blood pressure control and is especially important in controlling calcium entry into heart cells to trigger a regular heartbeat.	Lack of magnesium increases the risk of developing hypertension and increases the likelihood of spasms in the coronary arteries (linked with angina and heart attack). Magnesium supplements can reduce blood pressure by 2.7/3.4 mmHg if you have mild to moderate hypertension.	*300 mg daily* Take with food to maximize absorption. Magnesium citrate is most readily absorbed; magnesium gluconate is less likely to cause side-effects such as diarrhea at higher doses. Ensure you have a good calcium intake if you take magnesium.

SUPPLEMENT	RESEARCH FINDINGS	DOSE AND COMMENT
l-carnitine An amino acid needed to regulate fat metabolism in exercising muscles, such as the heart muscle. L-carnitine levels are reduced in people with hypertension.	Helps minimize heart damage in those at risk of a heart attack. Almost a quarter of men taking L-carnitine for 4 weeks became free of exercise-induced angina. It can also reduce pain on walking in those with hardening of the peripheral arteries.	*100–600 mg daily* L-carnitine is often combined with alpha lipoic acid (see page 89) in a 1:1 ratio. Doses of up to 2g daily are well tolerated.
Bilberry A rich source of anthocyanins—the pigments that give bilberries their blue color. Also rich in flavonoid glycosides; both have antioxidant and anti-inflammatory actions.	Strengthens and stabilizes blood vessels; reduces permeability of the blood-brain barrier in hypertension; inhibits unwanted blood clotting and reduces the risk of stroke. Especially important for people with hypertension-related eye damage.	*50–500 mg daily* Choose a product that is standardized (see page 48) to 25 percent anthocyanins. Take bilberry fruit extracts rather than leaf extracts.
Folic acid This is the more easily absorbed, synthetic form of the naturally occurring vitamin folate. Together with vitamin B12, it lowers homocysteine levels (see pages 20–30).	Can reduce elevated homocysteine levels by 25 percent. Taking it with vitamin B12 can produce a further 7 percent reduction. Folic acid improves baroreceptor sensitivity (see page 15).	*400–1,000 mcg daily* Folic acid is usually taken with 50 mcg vitamin B12, partly because they work in conjunction with one another and partly to avoid the masking of B12 deficiency anaemia.
Garlic Provides allicin, a powerful antioxidant.	In people with hypertension garlic can reduce systolic blood pressure by an average of 8 percent and diastolic blood pressure by 12 percent within 12 weeks. It also lowers LDL-cholesterol and triglyceride levels. It reduces blood stickiness, dilates blood vessels, and improves blood flow to the peripheral arteries.	*500–1,500 mg daily* Choose tablets standardized to provide 1,000–1,500mcg allicin (see page 48). Also choose a product that has an enteric coating—this can reduce the garlic odor on your breath and protect the active ingredients from degradation in the stomach.

SUPPLEMENT	RESEARCH FINDINGS	DOSE AND COMMENT
Calcium A mineral that plays a vital role in muscle contraction, nerve conduction, blood clotting, energy production, and the regulation of metabolic enzymes. The metabolism of calcium is disturbed in hypertension. Taking calcium supplements is advisable for anyone on a low-sodium diet.	Promotes sodium excretion, which helps lower blood pressure. Calcium supplements can reduce average blood pressure over a 24-hour period by 1.9/1.3 mmHg. Low intakes of calcium are linked with hypertension and stroke.	*500–1,000 mg daily* Take a calcium supplement with essential fatty acids if you have a tendency towards kidney stones (but seek medical advice first). Calcium lactate, calcium gluconate, calcium malate, and calcium citrate are the most readily absorbed supplements. Bear in mind that, if you are taking a calcium channel blocker drug, the blood pressure-lowering effect of calcium supplements is lost.
Reishi mushroom In China this is known as the "mushroom of immortality". Its Latin name is *Ganoderma lucidum*.	Reduces blood clotting, lowers blood pressure and LDL cholesterol, and reduces abnormal blood clotting. Contains substances that lower both diastolic and systolic blood pressure in a dose-dependent manner by inhibiting angiotensin-converting enzyme (ACE; see page 34).	*500–1,500 mg daily* If you are taking immunosuppressive drugs, anticoagulants or cholesterol-lowering medication, you should use reishi only under medical supervision.
Probiotics These are live, lactic acid-producing bacteria (for example, *Lactobacillis acidophilus*).	In one study, taking probiotic tablets (12g daily) for 4 weeks lowered blood pressure, by 3.2/5 mmHg in people with normal to high blood pressure, and by 11.2/6.5 mmHg in those with mild hypertension (compared with people who took an inactive placebo).	Select a supplement that supplies 1–2 billion colony-forming units (CFU) per dose.

SUPPLEMENT	RESEARCH FINDINGS	DOSE AND COMMENT
Omega-3 fish oil Contains the essential fatty acids: docosahexaenoic acid (DHA) and eicosapentanoic acid (EPA), which are derived from the microalgae on which fish feed. Vitamin E is added to supplements to protect fish oils from oxidation (rancidity). Supplementation is important if you are taking a beta-blocker (see page 33), as this drug lowers natural levels of EPA.	Maintains a regular heart rhythm, increases the elasticity of arteries, reduces blood stickiness and reduces blood triglyceride levels by 41 percent. Among 11,300 heart attack survivors, those taking supplements had a 15 percent lower risk of heart attack and stroke, and a 30 percent lower risk of cardiovascular death over three and a half years compared with those not taking supplements.	*300–900 mg omega-3s daily* (for example, obtained from 1g fish oil capsules, each supplying 180 mg EPA + 120 mg DHA) Choose emulsified oils to prevent the side-effect of unpleasant belching. Precautions: taking fish oils may affect diabetes control. Seek medical advice if you take a blood-thinning drug such as warfarin.

LIFESTYLE APPROACHES TO TREATMENT

Just about every healthcare professional and complementary therapist will recommend, alongside your main form of treatment for hypertension, you assess your diet and lifestyle and make changes if you need to. Health guidelines from around the world suggest you should:

- Keep your caffeine intake within acceptable limits. In particular, minimize your intake of coffee and cola (see pages 93–95).
- If you smoke, quit—or at least cut down.
- Limit the amount of alcohol you drink to two drinks or fewer per day (see pages 97–99).
- Avoid excessive amounts of stress.
- Introduce rest and relaxation into your life, so when stress affects you, you can deal with it.

- Do regular exercise—perform 30 to 45 minutes of aerobic exercise on most days of the week (see pages 100–102).
- Lose weight if you need to. Maintain an ideal body weight with a body mass index (BMI) of between 18.5–24.9 (see pages 102–105).

Collectively, these suggestions are known as lifestyle modifications. Although they might sound simple, in practice they can be among the hardest to achieve. Most people are able to make significant changes to the way they eat, such as increasing their intake of fruit and vegetables and cutting back on salt. Increasing your level of physical activity—and maintaining it—tends to be less simple. And among the most notoriously difficult habits to break are smoking and drinking too much alcohol.

Despite the fact that they pose a challenge, lifestyle modifications are very important—both for people with hypertension and for those at risk of developing it. Changes such as losing weight or quitting smoking can be the most powerful and positive things you do to improve your health and longevity.

If these lifestyle approaches to treatment sound daunting, please don't be put off—my aim in the programs in the next section (see pages 106–236), is to show you how to make sustainable changes in straightforward, enjoyable ways, no matter how fit—or unfit—you are at the moment.

LIMITING CAFFEINE

Caffeine is a natural stimulant found in some drinks and many over-the-counter drugs, especially those for headaches and colds. The amount of caffeine in a cup of coffee is about 70 mg, but can be as high as 150 mg if the coffee grounds are brewed for a long time. The average caffeine content of a cup of tea is significantly less: 40 mg per cup of black tea; 20 mg per cup of green tea; and 15 mg per cup of white tea.

THE EFFECTS OF CAFFEINE

Caffeine is a stimulant that mimics the effects of stress hormones: it increases your heart rate, raises your blood pressure and adrenaline levels, reduces your metabolism of glucose, and acts on your central nervous system to increase alertness and decrease your perception of effort and fatigue. The extent to which your blood pressure rises in response to a cup of coffee depends on how accustomed you are to caffeine. If you're an infrequent caffeine consumer, two cups of coffee can increase your blood pressure by 5 mmHg. If you're a habitual caffeine consumer, individual cups of coffee don't cause the same sudden rise in blood pressure, but this might be because your blood pressure is persistently raised by caffeine anyway.

Everyone metabolizes caffeine at a different rate. The average time taken to metabolize half a given caffeine dose is around four hours, with a range of two to ten hours. Some people metabolize it slowly and get irritable and jittery, while others can drink lots of coffee with no side-effects. The rate at which caffeine is cleared from your system is reduced if you have also been drinking alcohol. A person weighing 154 pounds, for example, who drinks more than six cups of coffee a day is at risk of caffeine poisoning, with symptoms that can include tremors, nausea, palpitations, anxiety, panic attacks, and confusion.

Caffeine is also addictive, in the sense that you become tolerant to it and have to drink more and more to achieve the same stimulant effect. If you stop a high intake of caffeine suddenly, you can have withdrawal

HOW CAFFEINE AFFECTS YOU

Try this simple test to assess the effects of caffeine on your blood pressure. Make your usual cup of coffee but, rather than drinking it straight away, wait for 10 minutes. Spend this time reading a book or listening to music—or doing any activity that helps you to relax. Now check your resting blood pressure using a home monitoring device (see page 31). Drink your coffee and check your blood pressure at 10-minute intervals for the next hour to see whether or not your caffeine intake affects your blood pressure.

symptoms such as headaches, fatigue, sweating, anxiety, and muscle pains—these typically last for around 36 hours.

CUTTING DOWN ON CAFFEINE

If you have hypertension, it's worth minimizing your caffeine intake. If you drink many cups of coffee or a lot of cola every day, cut down by one caffeinated drink a day to avoid withdrawal symptoms. Try to switch slowly to decaffeinated brands and make coffee less strong by brewing grounds for a shorter length of time, or by using fewer instant granules. Alternatively, try switching to green or white tea. This provides a lower level of caffeine plus beneficial antioxidants. The benefits of tea drinking outweigh the adverse effects of caffeine—evidence suggests tea can protect against coronary heart disease. Herbal teas such as rooibos are also good—rooibos is made from a South African shrub and is high in antioxidants.

QUITTING SMOKING

Smoking reduces the amount of oxygen in your blood; it makes your blood more sticky and prone to clotting; and it damages your arteries. In the long term it increases your risk of hypertension by at least 30 percent and your risk of coronary heart disease seven-fold. It also quadruples your risk of having a stroke.

THE EFFECTS OF SMOKING

Every time you smoke a cigarette, your blood pressure can rise by 9/8 mmHg. If you both smoke a cigarette and drink coffee, the increase is even greater and, in some people, is as high as 21/17 mmHg. (Nicotine replacement products are, therefore, not a good idea if you have uncontrolled hypertension.)

In the long term, chemicals in cigarette smoke damage the linings of your artery walls, causing inflammation that hastens the hardening and furring up of the arteries (and makes hypertension worse). Long-term smokers tend to have thicker, less elastic arteries, and enlargement of the left ventricle of the heart. Smoking has also been shown to increase the risk of poor kidney function. In addition, people who smoke and have hypertension tend to require more drugs to control their hypertension. This is because smoking reduces the effectiveness of anti-hypertensive drugs, especially beta-blockers and angiotensin II blockers.

If you smoke, consider taking pycnogenol—extracts from the bark of the French maritime pine. A dose of 125 mg pycnogenol is as effective in preventing susceptibility to blood clots in smokers as 500 mg aspirin, but without the stomach irritation that aspirin causes.

STOPPING SMOKING

The benefits of stopping smoking are soon realized. Within eight hours, levels of oxygen in your circulation increase; within 48 hours, the stickiness of your blood reduces, and within three months your peripheral circulation significantly improves.

Find support to help you quit—stopping smoking is easier if you do it with a friend or relative. Focus on getting through each day—try not to think long term, as this can be daunting. Keep your hands busy with activities, such as drawing, painting, origami, knitting, embroidery, or home-handyman work—psychologists have found the hand-to-mouth habit is one of the things that makes quitting smoking so difficult. Increasing the amount of exercise you do will help to curb withdrawal symptoms by increasing secretion of opium-like endorphins. It's also important to identify situations in which you used to smoke and either avoid them or plan coping strategies in advance. For example, you could practice saying: "No thanks, I've stopped" or "No thanks, I'm cutting down."

WATCH YOUR WEIGHT

When you quit smoking make sure you don't experience a subsequent increase in your weight and waist measurements—this may offset the expected decrease in your risk of coronary heart disease and stroke. See pages 102–105 for advice about achieving and maintaining a healthy weight.

To help overcome nicotine cravings, try sucking on an artificial cigarette or herbal stick; do 30 minutes of brisk exercise; take a flower remedy (such as rescue remedy); or try essential oil products designed to reduce cravings. All these aids are available from pharmacies. If you do use nicotine replacement products to help you quit, monitor your blood pressure closely.

LIMITING ALCOHOL

In small quantities alcohol has a beneficial effect on blood pressure in that it acts as a diuretic and increases sodium loss. Alcohol also increases levels of beneficial HDL-cholesterol and lowers harmful LDL-cholesterol (see pages 72–73). Red wine is particularly beneficial for people with hypertension because it's rich in antioxidants and offers protection against coronary heart disease. As a result, drinking up to ⅔ cup red wine a day is recommended—you'll notice that I include a glass of red wine in the eating plans in Part Three. If you prefer not to drink alcohol, unsweetened red grape juice provides the same antioxidant benefits, thanks to the phytochemicals present in the grapes.

ADVERSE EFFECTS OF ALCOHOL

If you have three or more drinks a day, the benefits of alcohol start to reverse. A high alcohol intake leads to sodium retention, and increases your resistance to the hormone insulin, both of which contribute to hypertension. Above an intake of three drinks (1 ounce alcohol) per day, every additional drink (⅓ ounce alcohol) increases your average systolic blood pressure by 1–2 mmHg, and diastolic blood pressure by 1 mmHg. Excess alcohol also affects your heart (leading to irregular heart rhythms and cardiac enlargement) and your liver (leading to fibrosis and cirrhosis). Excessive alcohol intake is most harmful when it occurs without food. Women are more susceptible to the adverse effects of excessive alcohol than men. Even if you haven't had an alcoholic drink for several days, avoid binge drinking.

If you are overweight (see pages 102–105), you need to monitor your alcohol intake carefully. Being overweight or obese can worsen hypertension and increase your risk of cardiovascular problems. Alcohol is a source of extra calories in your diet—a glass of dry white or red wine contains about 90 calories (sweet white wine contains more), as does a glass (8 ounces) of beer. A shot measure of hard liquor, such as whiskey, gin, or vodka, contains about 50 calories—and significantly more if you mix it with a sugary mixer such as cola, lemonade, or tonic.

REDUCING YOUR ALCOHOL INTAKE

If you drink more than ⅔ ounce alcohol per day, aim to cut down. Each drink you forgo will lower both your systolic and diastolic blood pressure by about 1 mmHg. To work out your daily alcohol consumption, ⅓ ounce alcohol is equivalent to:

- 1¼ cups beer.
- Scant ½ cup wine.
- 2 tablespoons sherry.
- A shot of hard liquor.

If you are a very heavy drinker, ask your doctor to help you start drinking less—stopping abruptly can cause your blood pressure to rise. If you are a light to moderate drinker, try the following suggestions:

- Put your glass down between sips.
- Savor each sip, holding it longer in your mouth.
- Alternate alcoholic and nonalcoholic drinks.
- Choose unsweetened fruit juices or nonalcoholic cocktails, such as mango juice with coconut milk.
- Try sparkling mineral water with lime juice.
- Try tonic water with a dash of Angostura bitters instead of gin.
- Mix chilled wine with sparkling mineral water for a refreshing spritzer.
- Elderflower cordial diluted with mineral water makes a great substitute for white wine.

- An herb known as kudzu (Japanese arrowroot), reduces alcohol cravings. Research suggests this action is due to substances known as isoflavones.

OVERCOMING STRESS

When you feel stressed, your body prepares for physical activity as part of its ancient flight or fight response. Nerve signals from your brain trigger the release of adrenaline (epinephrine), noradrenaline (norepinephrine), and cortisol from your adrenal glands, all of which increase blood pressure by constricting peripheral arteries. For ancient humans, this insured more blood was pumped to the muscles and brain (for fighting and fleeing), and it minimized blood loss as a result of wounds. After the battle was fought (or ancient humans had run away), blood pressure returned to normal.

In modern life, however, stress rarely results in fighting or fleeing, and the affects of adrenaline, noradrenaline, and cortisol can persist in the circulation over prolonged periods of time. In susceptible individuals this results in overactivity of the sympathetic nervous system as part of the stress response. Instead of short-lived rises in blood pressure, stress causes blood pressure to become persistently raised.

COMBATING STRESS

I advise everyone, with or without hypertension, to take steps to reduce their exposure to stress or to find strategies for dealing with it. Here are some suggestions that everyone can try:

- Stop what you are doing and inwardly say "calm" to yourself. Combine this with the following step.
- Take a deep breath in and let it out slowly, concentrating on the movement of your diaphragm. Do this two or three times until you feel more in control.
- If you're sitting down, stand up and gently stretch to your fullest possible extent. Shake your hands and arms briskly, then shrug your shoulders.

WHITE-COAT HYPERTENSION

Stress is linked with white-coat hypertension, in which blood pressure goes up and down significantly over relatively short periods of time during the day. White-coat hypertension is a strong predictor of future hypertension. It's also associated with poor function of the left ventricle of the heart and decreased elasticity and increased stiffness of the artery walls. White-coat hypertension is diagnosed if your blood pressure suddenly becomes high when measured (usually by someone wearing a white coat) in a stressful situation, such as a doctor's surgery or hospital (see page 27).

- Go for a brisk walk, even if it's only briefly around the room. Regular brisk, noncompetitive exercise is one of the best ways to lower stress hormones.
- Go somewhere private and groan or shout as loudly as you want. Some people find it helpful to punch a soft cushion as hard as possible.
- Place a few drops of a flower essence, such as rescue remedy, under your tongue.
- Listen to calming background music—natural sounds like recordings of the sea, bird songs, a babbling brook, or a waterfall are ideal.
- Organize your life, make comprehensive lists, and manage your time more effectively—prioritize tasks so you can deal with pressures one at a time. Where possible, try to delegate to others.
- Say "no" to unreasonable demands.
- Make a point of complimenting those around you—making others feel good will make you feel good.
- Watch a comedy or do something that makes you laugh—laughter is a great antidote to stress.
- Use visualization or meditation to find calm.

GETTING REGULAR EXERCISE

We now know regular aerobic exercise has profound benefits for the cardiovascular system. Among other things, it lowers raised blood pressure and reduces the risk of premature death from coronary heart disease by more than 40 percent.

HOW MUCH EXERCISE?

Studies suggest that it's wise to exercise every day. Physical activity doesn't need to be intense. Brisk walking for 30 to 60 minutes a day, most days, produces significant benefits for people with hypertension. In fact, activities such as doing home improvements, gardening, and dancing—anything that leaves you feeling warm and slightly out of breath—are as effective as swimming or cycling for cardiovascular health. Yoga and qigong (see pages 58–63) are good for bringing balance, equilibrium, and relaxation.

Researchers have found that aerobic exercise doesn't have to take place in a single session—two or three daily sessions of 10 to 15 minutes are just as good.

EXERCISING AT THE RIGHT INTENSITY

Try to exercise briskly enough to raise your pulse above 100 beats per minute, raise a light sweat and make you slightly breathless—but not so briskly that you cannot hold a conversation. Measuring your pulse rate during exercise will insure you stay within the safe range for burning

10-SECOND PULSE RANGES	
Age group	Pulse range
20–29	20–27
30–39	19–25
40–49	18–23
50–59	17–22
60–69	16–21
70+	15–20

excess fat and improving cardiovascular fitness without overstressing your heart.

Take your 10-second pulse every 10 minutes or so as you exercise. Simply look at your watch and count the number of pulses you feel during a 10-second period. Your pulse is most easily felt on the inner side of your wrist on the same side as your thumb or on the side of your neck, just under your jaw.

If you are unfit, make sure your pulse stays at the lower end of your 10-second pulse range at first, then slowly work up to the upper end over several weeks. Consult the chart above to find the recommended 10-second pulse range for your age.

If at any time your pulse rate goes higher than it should, stop exercising and walk around slowly until your pulse falls. At the end of 20 minutes' exercise, you should feel invigorated rather than exhausted.

EXERCISING SAFELY

Warm up and cool down before and after any form of exercise with a few simple bends and stretches. This helps to avoid muscle injuries, and pain and stiffness. For comfort, wear loose clothing and footwear specifically designed for the exercise you have chosen. Don't exercise straight after a heavy meal, after drinking alcohol, or if you feel unwell. Stop exercising immediately if you feel very short of breath or unwell. If you are taking medication, seek medical advice before starting an exercise program.

MAINTAINING A HEALTHY WEIGHT

If you have hypertension, losing a relatively small amount of excess fat will significantly lower your blood pressure. If you combine exercise with losing weight, the blood pressure-lowering effect is even greater.

ASSESSING YOUR WEIGHT

Your weight is usually assessed using the body mass index (BMI), but another factor to take into account is where you store fat—on your hips or on your waist. Fat deposits on your waist are associated with an increased risk of cardiovascular problems.

BODY MASS INDEX

According to the World Health Organization, if your BMI is 18.5 or under, you're underweight; if it's between 18.5–24.9 your weight is ideal; if it's between 25–29.9, you're overweight; 30 or above, you're obese; and over 40, you're morbidly obese. Calculate your BMI using the formula described below. (Please note that BMI values are less accurate if you're very muscly or frail—ask your doctor.) You can also assess whether you are a healthy weight by consulting the chart on the opposite page.

WAIST SIZE

If you store excess fat around your waist in an apple-shape, you're twice as likely to develop hypertension and coronary heart disease as someone who is pear-shaped, with excess fat around their hips.

Having a waist size between 32 to 35 inches for women, or 37 to 40 inches for men, carries a similar health risk as a BMI of 25 to 30—it means you are overweight and increases your risk of heart disease by a factor of 1.5. Women with a waist circumference larger than 35 inches and men with a waist circumference larger than 40 inches have an even greater risk of heart disease.

CALCULATING BMI

You need two measurements: your weight in pounds and your height in inches.
For example, 150 pounds and 68 inches.

↓

Multiply your weight by 703. For example: 150 x 703 = 105,450
Divide the answer by your height: 105,450 ÷ 68 = 1,550

↓

Divide that answer by your height again: 1,550 ÷ 68 = 22.8
This is your BMI, which allows you to assess how healthy your weight is.

Waist size reductions of just 2 to 4 inches can significantly lower your blood pressure and reduce your risk of a future heart attack.

LOSING EXCESS WEIGHT

If you're overweight, try to lose weight slowly and steadily until you reach the healthy range for your height. If you manage this, you should notice significant reductions in your blood pressure and, if you are on anti-hypertensive medication, your doctor may be able to reduce the dose and/or number of anti-hypertensive drugs you are taking.

The best way to lose weight permanently is controversial. In the past, healthy eating messages have consistently recommended low-fat diets to reduce the incidence of obesity and coronary heart disease. Unfortunately, research shows that low-fat diets can lower the level of healthy HDL-cholesterol and increase the level of unhealthy LDL-cholesterol in your body, which can, in turn, increase the risk of coronary heart disease.

In contrast, a number of studies suggest that following a low-carbohydrate diet can promote weight loss, lower hypertension by 1–10 mmHg and reduce LDL-cholesterol and triglycerides, while raising HDL-cholesterol and improving blood glucose control.

Extremely low carbohydrate diets such as the Atkins diet do not suit everyone. In my opinion, the ideal compromise appears to be a low-glycemic diet, in which carbohydrates that produce rapid increases in blood glucose levels are avoided (see pages 77–80). This makes sense, as carbohydrates increase the secretion of insulin—the main fat-storing hormone in the body. Most people with hypertension will benefit from cutting back on carbohydrates, especially if they also tend to store fat around their waist.

When you follow my eating plans in the programs in the next part of the book, you should be able to lose weight slowly over a period of weeks and months. This means that instead of dieting to achieve weight loss, you adopt new, healthier eating habits—ones you will be able to sustain in the long term, and ones that will enable you to keep weight off permanently.

THE HEALTHY WEIGHT FOR YOUR HEIGHT

FEET	POUNDS
4' 10"	88–118 lb.
4' 11"	92–123 lb.
5 ft.	94–126 lb.
5' 1"	98–131 lb.
5' 2"	100–135 lb.
5' 3"	104–140 lb.
5' 4"	108–145 lb.
5' 5"	111–147 lb.
5' 6"	115–154 lb.
5' 7"	118–159 lb.
5' 8"	122–164 lb.
5' 9	117–168 lb.
5' 10"	129–173 lb.
15' 11"	132–177 lb.
6 ft.	136–183 lb.
6' 1"	139–187 lb.
6' 2"	144–193 lb.
6' 3"	147–197 lb.
6' 4"	152–204 lb.

PART THREE

THE NATURAL HEALTH GURU PROGRAMS

Having explained what high blood pressure is in Part One, and how it can be treated naturally in Part Two, Part Three offers you the tools to transform your life. First, I ask you to complete a questionnaire (see pages 109–111). Your answers will help to identify the best program for you as an individual: the gentle, moderate, or full-strength program. The gentle program is aimed at people who know they have diet and lifestyle issues to address. It offers you an eating plan that supplies nutritious foods that will benefit your health. The moderate program is aimed at people who want to enhance an already healthy diet and lifestyle. The full-strength program incorporates all the superfoods research suggests have the most powerful effect on hypertension—this program is designed to achieve the greatest result in the least amount of time. Each program supplies daily menu plans, healthy salt-free recipes, daily exercise routines, and suggestions for therapies you can try at home. Each program lasts 14 days, but can be repeated so it lasts for 28 days in total. Once you have followed a program, you should notice significant changes in your blood pressure and overall well-being. You can then choose to continue with the diet and lifestyle principles outlined in your program, or you can move onto the next program.

THE NATURAL HEALTH GURU QUESTIONNAIRE

Before you start on the programs in this section of the book, I'd like you to answer the questions on the next three pages. Your answers will give you an overview of your current health, diet, and lifestyle habits, and help you to decide which is the best program to start with. Whereas a fit 35-year-old with borderline hypertension might be able to start on the full-strength program, an overweight 70-year-old on several medications for hypertension will be better off with the gentle program, at least at first. Age isn't always an indicator of health and fitness, however. A very overweight 30-year-old, who rarely exercises and eats lots of fast food should start with the gentle program, despite his or her age. Likewise, a slim, fit grandmother of 70 years, with an adventurous approach to life might be able to start on the moderate program.

Answer either A, B, or C to each of the 30 questions—whichever seems the closest to your ideal response. If you answer:

- Mostly As: it's a good idea to start with the gentle program.
- Mostly Bs: you might wish to start on the moderate program.
- Mostly Cs: you can follow the full-strength program.

All three programs are based on the principles of the DASH diet (see page 66) and encourage you to eat plenty of fruit and vegetables and whole grains, and cut down your intake of salt, sugar, and unhealthy fats. The gentle program consists of foods that will be familiar to you and includes a small amount of red meat. In the moderate and full-strength programs, I encourage you to adopt an increasingly vegetarian or fish-based diet, and to eat more of the superfoods that are beneficial for hypertension. I also suggest sprouting your own beans and seeds and making your own fruit and vegetable juices in the moderate and full-strength programs.

The amount of daily exercise I recommend in the programs varies from 15 to 20 minutes in the gentle program to 30 to 45 minutes in the full-strength program. Although it might be tempting to start on the full-strength program right away (because it provides the most benefits), it's unwise to do this if you answer mostly As. It's more beneficial to begin gently and build up over time so your body becomes accustomed to the changes in your diet and activity levels.

Another way of tackling the programs is to do each one in turn, regardless of your current health and lifestyle: if you opt for this approach, begin with the gentle program, then work your way up to the moderate and the full-strength programs. This provides you with three months of menu plans and exercise routines.

If you're taking any prescribed medications, or if you are pregnant, or planning to be, seek medical advice from your doctor before embarking on major dietary and lifestyle changes. If you have diabetes (Type 2 diabetes and hypertension are often associated), you will need to monitor your blood glucose closely as you change your diet and activity levels.

1 How old are you?
  A 50 years or older
  B 30–50 years
  C 30 years or under

2 Do you have hypertension?
  A Yes
  B Borderline hypertension
  C No, but it runs in my family

3 Are you currently taking medication for hypertension?
  A Yes, I'm taking more than one anti-hypertensive drug
  B Yes, I'm on one anti-hypertensive drug
  C No

4 Are you overweight?
  A Yes, I need to lose at least 14 lb
  B Yes, I need to lose less than 14 lb)
  C No, I'm in the healthy weight range for my height

5 Do you tend to store fat around your waist and tummy rather than your hips?
  A Yes, I'm apple-shaped
  B No, I'm pear shaped
  C No, but beer bellies run in my family

6 Do you have diabetes?
  A Yes
  B No, but diabetes runs in my family
  C No, and I have no family history of diabetes

7 Do you have high cholesterol levels?
  A Yes
  B No, but cholesterol problems run
     in my family
  C No

8 Have you ever had a heart attack?
  A Yes
  B No, but heart attacks run in
     my family
  C No, and I have no family history
     of heart attacks

9 Have you ever had a stroke?
  A Yes
  B No, but strokes run in my family
  C No, and I have no family history
     of strokes

10 What is your resting heart rate?
   (Skip this question if you are taking
   a beta-blocker drug.)
  A 80 beats per minute or more
  B 70–80 beats per minute
  C Fewer than 70 beats per minute

11 Do you smoke cigarettes?
  A Yes (but I'm trying to quit)
  B I used to, but quit in the past
     five years
  C No

12 How much alcohol do you drink?
  A Women: more than 14 drinks per week
     Men: more than 21 drinks per week
  B Women: 14 drinks per week or fewer
     Men: 21 drinks per week or fewer
  C None or very little

13 How many caffeinated drinks, such as
   coffee or cola, do you drink a day?
  A More than 6
  B Between 3 and 6
  C 2 or fewer

14 Do you regularly feel you are under a lot
   of stress?
  A Yes, all the time
  B Yes, once or twice a week
  C No, I'm quite laid back

15 Do you regularly feel anxious or panicky?
  A Yes, virtually all the time
  B Yes, several times a week
  C No, only occasionally

16 How often do you experience
   headaches?
  A Several times a week
  B Occasionally
  C Hardly ever

17 Do you feel that you lack energy or are
   exhausted?
  A Yes, regularly
  B Occasionally
  C No, not at all

18 How often do you exercise (or have a
   high level of physical activity; for
   example, gardening)?
  A I have not yet managed to fit regular
     exercise into my life
  B I exercise for 30 minutes 2 or 3 times
     a week
  C I exercise for at least 30 minutes on
     at least 5 days a week

19 Are you a vegetarian?
   A No
   B No, but I regularly have days in which
     I don't eat meat
   C Yes

20 On how many days of the week do you
   eat meat?
   A Every day or most days
   B Several days
   C One day or fewer

21 How often do you eat processed and
   pre-packaged foods?
   A Most days
   B Several times a week
   C I rarely/never touch them

22 How often do you eat fast food?
   A Several times a week
   B Around once a week
   C I rarely/never touch them

23 How often do you eat fried foods?
   A Several times a week
   B Around once a week
   C I rarely/never touch them

24 Do you eat at least 8 portions of fruit/
   vegetables a day?
   A No, I eat fewer than 8
   B Yes, I eat at least 8
   C Yes, I usually eat more than 8

25 How often do you eat fish?
   A Hardly ever
   B At least once or twice a week
   C Three or more times a week, or I take
     a daily fish oil supplement

26 How often do you add salt to your food?
   A I always add salt during cooking, and
     add salt to my food at the table
   B I've stopped adding salt during
     cooking, but sometimes add it at
     the table
   C I do not add any salt to my food, and
     I check labels for sodium content

27 Do you follow a low-fat diet?
   A Not really
   B Yes, I've switched to low-fat products
     for example, milk
   C Yes, I always check labels for fat
     content

28 Do you eat a low-sugar diet?
   A Not really
   B Yes, I've cut right back on candy
     and snacks
   C Yes, I always check labels for sugar
     content

29 Would you describe yourself as an
   adventurous eater?
   A No, not at all
   B I try to eat at least one new dish
     each week
   C Yes, definitely

30 Are you willing to change the way you
   eat significantly?
   A I'll start gently and see how I go
   B Yes, I want to make a difference
     without going wild
   C Yes, whatever it takes

STARTING THE PROGRAMS

Now you have decided which program is right for you, you can set a date on which to start. Give yourself a few days to read through the program and gather the things you need. You will need to go food shopping and buy items, such as essential oils and supplements, as well as book appointments with complementary therapists.

Make a copy of the chart below and fill in your statistics at the beginning and end of each program. Seeing improvements and benefits presented in a tangible way can act as a powerful motivator to continue with the diet and lifestyle changes you have made.

Although you can go to your doctor or a pharmacist for a blood pressure reading, I strongly advise you to invest in a home blood pressure monitoring device. Before you start a program, measure your blood pressure regularly throughout the day for a couple of days—calculate the average reading and enter this in the chart below.

I have also allowed space for you to enter your cholesterol, triglyceride, and homocysteine (see pages 29 and 72) levels. The levels of fats and homocysteine in your blood are a strong indicator of how healthy your cardiovascular system is—and how likely you are to develop coronary heart disease. If your levels decrease, as I would expect, this really helps to underline how much your dietary and lifestyle changes are improving your health. Your doctor should be happy to arrange these tests for you.

PROGRESS CHART FOR ALL PROGRAMS

MEASUREMENT	START DATE	FINISH DATE	IMPROVEMENT
Weight			minus
Blood pressure			minus
Total cholesterol			minus
LDL-cholesterol			minus
HDL-cholesterol			plus
Triglycerides			minus
Homocysteine			minus

INTRODUCING THE GENTLE PROGRAM

The gentle program aims to ease you into diet, exercise, and lifestyle changes as painlessly as possible. It provides 14 daily plans you can repeat to create a program lasting for 28 days. It might take a while to settle into the program but, once you get accustomed to the diet and lifestyle changes, feel free to make your own adjustments that take into account your personal likes, dislikes, and lifestyle.

THE GENTLE PROGRAM DIET

The daily food plans in the gentle program should not be radically different from your current way of eating. They are designed to introduce you to a lower glycemic index (GI) diet (see pages 77–80) with less refined carbohydrate than you might be used to. The diet also follows the principles of the Dietary Approaches to Stop Hypertension (DASH; see page 66), in which the emphasis is on fruit, vegetables, saladstuff, nuts, whole grains, poultry, fish, and low-fat dairy products.

This approach increases your intake of fiber, antioxidants (especially carotenoids), vitamins (including folate), minerals (such as potassium, magnesium, and calcium), and monounsaturated and omega-3 fats. It reduces your intake of sodium, saturated fat, trans fats, and cholesterol. Research suggests this has the potential to lower your blood pressure by 4/2–7/4 mmHg or more within 30 days, even if you're taking anti-hypertensive medications (various trials show that DASH enhances the effects of prescribed drugs).

In addition to lowering blood pressure, the gentle program diet might also lower your total and LDL-cholesterol and your triglyceride levels (see pages 72–73). People who are older, and those who previously had high intakes of salt (sodium chloride) are likely to experience the greatest benefits from the gentle program.

If you wish, you can have one 5-ounce glass of red wine per day during the gentle program. Research shows that a daily glass of red wine can reduce the risk of coronary heart disease by one-third. If you prefer to avoid alcohol, you can have a glass of unsweetened red grape juice

SHOPPING LIST

These are items that I suggest you buy on a regular basis. They are featured in the suggested meals for the next 14 days. Whenever possible, buy regularly in small quantities for optimum freshness.

DRINKS

almond and soymilk; black, green, or white tea; fruit and herbal teas; mineral water (low sodium); red and white (dry) wine; unsweetened fruit juices (or fresh produce for home juicing)

DAIRY PRODUCTS

plain low-fat cottage cheese, plain low-fat fromage blanc, plain low-fat yogurt with live cultures, mozzarella cheese, omega-3 enriched spread, 1% or 2% milk

FRUIT AND VEGETABLES

organic fruit: apples, bananas, berries, cherries, figs, grapes, kiwi, lemons, limes, mango, melon, nectarines, oranges, papaya, peaches, pears, pineapple, red grapefruit (see caution on page 120), star fruit
organic vegetables: bok choy, broccoli, cabbage, carrots, Chinese broccoli, corn kernels, corn on the cob, eggplant, green beans, leeks, mushrooms, onions, peas, potatoes (waxy, new), red cabbage, shallots, snow peas, spinach, sweet potatoes, zucchini
organic salad ingredients: arugula, avocados, beansprouts, bell peppers, celery, cucumber, iceberg lettuce, peppers, salad leaves, scallions, tomatoes, watercress
dried fruit: apricots, dates, figs, raisins

NUTS AND SEEDS (UNSALTED)

almonds (whole, ground, and flaked); Brazil nuts; coconut; flax, pumpkin, sesame, and sunflower seeds; nut butter (such as almond); walnuts

HERBS, SPICES, OILS, VINEGAR

herbs: basil, bay leaf, chives, cilantro, garlic, mint, oregano, parsley, rosemary, tarragon, thyme
spices: black pepper, fresh chilies, ground cinnamon, coriander seeds, ground cumin, curry powder, gingerroot, nutmeg
oils and vinegar: extra virgin coconut oil, extra virgin olive oil, olive oil, walnut oil, balsamic vinegar, low-fat mayonnaise, low-sodium soy sauce, wholegrain mustard

GRAINS

brown rice; bulgur wheat; crispbread; instant oatmeal; muesli cereals (for example, barley, bran, rye, or wheat flakes—or buy unsweetened muesli); rice cakes; rolled oats; pita; rye bread; whole-grain bread/rolls; wholewheat pasta

PROTEINS

halibut, mackerel (fresh and smoked), salmon, trout (fresh and smoked), tuna (in spring water/olive oil), omega-3 rich eggs, lamb shanks, skinless chicken/turkey

MISCELLANEOUS

organic honey, organic dark chocolate (at least 70 percent cocoa solids)

instead. This provides the same heart-healthy antioxidants as red wine, and research suggests grape juice is at least as good as red wine in improving dilation of arteries. It does not have the same beneficial effect on cholesterol levels, however. You can also include a daily 1½-ounce piece of dark chocolate (at least 70 percent cocoa solids) during the gentle program.

FOODS TO AVOID OR EAT LESS OF

While on the gentle program it's important to avoid refined carbohydrates (for example, cakes, cookies, and sugary drinks), processed foods (for example, canned meat, and packages of soups), candies, and excess alcohol. These foods make hypertension worse—eliminating them and following a healthy eating plan can significantly bring your blood pressure down in a relatively short amount of time.

Begin the program by looking at the food labels on all cans, packages, and jars in your kitchen cupboards. Throw away all foods containing a lot of saturated fat, sodium or salt, or sugar. For guidelines about what constitutes a "lot" of these ingredients, see pages 75–77 and 80. Also throw away foods that contain trans fats (see page 73).

The gentle program diet encourages you to eat red meat in moderation. Long-term observational studies show that a higher intake of fruit and vegetables and a lower intake of red meat can prevent increases in blood pressure with age. The occasional lean steak or lamb shank is fine, but as the World Cancer Research Fund suggests, you should limit red meat intake to less than 3 ounces per day.

None of the recipes in the gentle program include table salt (sodium chloride). Instead, you can add flavor to food by using fresh herbs and black pepper. Initially food might taste bland, but over the course of the month you will start to notice how much better fresh, unsalted food can taste. Please do not be tempted to add salt during cooking or at the table; if you do, you will not gain the optimum benefits from this program.

LOSING WEIGHT

Although it's not specifically designed to be a weight-loss tool, the gentle program diet should enable you to lose any excess weight slowly and naturally. This is because you are eating healthily and avoiding high intakes of refined carbohydrates and excess fats, both of which contribute to excess weight and hypertension.

If you need to lose weight, you might wish to enhance the process by eating smaller portions and by cutting out some of the starchy foods suggested in each daily eating plan (for example, wholewheat toast, rolls, pasta, rice, and couscous). Make the focus of your diet protein foods, fruit, and vegetables.

GENTLE PROGRAM SUPPLEMENTS

I suggest you take the following supplements while you follow the gentle program. They are widely available in drug stores, supermarkets, and whole-food stores. You can find information about these supplements and their blood pressure-lowering effects on pages 86–92.

Recommended daily supplements
- Vitamin C (500 mg)
- Vitamin E (200 i.u/134 mg)
- Lycopene carotenoid complex (15 mg)
- Selenium (50 mcg)
- Coenzyme Q10 (60 mg)
- Garlic tablets (allicin yield 1,000–1,500 mcg)
- Omega-3 fish oil (300 mg daily; for example, 1 g fish oil capsule supplying 180 mg eicosapentaenoic acid, EPA, plus 120 mg docosahexaenoic acid, DHA)

Optional daily supplements (these will provide additional health benefits)
- Alpha-lipoic acid (100 mg). May be combined with L-carnitine in a 1:1 ratio
- Magnesium (300 mg)
- Calcium (500 mg)
- Folic acid (400 mcg) plus vitamin B12 (50 mcg)
- Reishi (500 mg)
- Bilberry fruit extracts (60 mg—standardized to give 25 percent anthocyanins)
- Probiotics (in the form of fermented milk drinks, live yogurt, or supplements)

THE GENTLE PROGRAM EXERCISE ROUTINE

If you have not exercised much over the past few years, it's important to ease into regular exercise slowly to avoid aches and pains that might otherwise put you off. These daily exercise routines provide a series of stretching exercises to help limber you up and get you moving. A regular morning stretch routine will help to tone your body and relax your mind—both of which can bring your blood pressure down.

In addition, you should do some cardiovascular exercise, such as walking, for at least 15 minutes a day. You need to exercise at a rate that is brisk enough to raise your pulse rate by about 100 beats per minute (unless you're taking a beta-blocker drug; see page 33) and to make you slightly breathless.

Over the next month, you will gradually build up your cardiovascular exercise in time and intensity until you are doing 30 minutes' brisk exercise every day. As explained on page 101, you don't have to do 30 minutes' exercise all in one go—you can do three bouts of 10 minutes each if you prefer.

Walking is one of the easiest, and cheapest, ways of achieving and maintaining fitness. It is useful to buy a small pedometer to clip to your clothes. This measures the number of steps you take each day. Ideally, you need to take 10,000 steps a day. If you are unfit, aim for 5,000 steps and slowly work up to a higher target.

When starting an exercise routine, always monitor your 10-second pulse rate (see pages 101–102) to insure you're not overexerting yourself. If you have angina or a history of heart attack, ask your doctor for guidance on how much exercise you can take.

THE GENTLE PROGRAM THERAPIES

I suggest a number of complementary therapies, such as meditation, that can reduce blood pressure. Some, such as relaxation therapies, can be practised alone at home, while others are practitioner-led, at least initially. Please look at days seven and fourteen of the program now so you can make appointments with the appropriate therapists.

THE GENTLE PROGRAM
DAY ONE

DAILY MENU

Breakfast: homemade muesli (see page 141) with almonds and blueberries

Morning snack: a piece of fruit (choose from the selection on the shopping list; see page 114)

Lunch: tuna, bean, and pepper salad (see page 144). Small wholewheat pita bread or mixed-grain roll

Afternoon snack: low-fat yogurt with live cultures. Handful of dried figs and almonds

Dinner: baked oriental salmon (see page 146). Brown rice. Bowl of mixed salad leaves

Drinks: 2½ cups 1% or 2% milk. Unsweetened fresh fruit juice. Unlimited green, black, white, or herbal tea, and mineral water. 5 ounces (⅔ cup) red wine or unsweetened red grape juice

Supplements: see page 116

DAILY EXERCISE ROUTINE

Over the next week, I introduce a gentle exercise routine that begins with the top of your body and works down. When you've mastered the whole routine, do it every morning when you get up. Today, do the following head/neck stretch, and go for a brisk 15 to 20-minute walk.

HEAD/NECK STRETCH

1 Stand comfortably with feet apart and shoulders relaxed.
2 Slowly drop your head toward your left shoulder. Hold the stretch for a count of five.
3 Repeat on the right side.

AROMATHERAPY

During this first week of the program, I introduce a range of relaxing

REMEMBER YOUR SUPPLEMENTS
Keep your supplements in the same place as your other medication. Set the alarm on a watch or cell phone to remind you to take them. Pill containers divided into seven sections (one for every day of the week) are also useful. Fill one up every Sunday. Keep medicines away from children.

ways to harness the therapeutic effects of aromatherapy. You will try soothing essential oils with sedative properties that promote a good night's sleep. Sleep is important—research suggests people with hypertension who lie awake at night have a higher blood pressure and pulse rate, and are at greater risk of heart damage than those who sleep well. Tonight, at bedtime, put 4 drops of pure lavender essential oil on a tissue and tuck it under your pillow. Alternatively, use a lavender pillow or pozy containing dried lavender. Lavender essential oil is gentle and suits most people.

DAY TWO

DAILY MENU

Breakfast: one red grapefruit, fresh or lightly broiled (see box, overleaf). Wholewheat toast with a scraping of omega-3 enriched spread or butter **Morning snack:** a piece of fruit **Lunch:** coronation turkey salad with cranberries (see page 144). Low-fat yogurt with live cultures with fresh fruit **Afternoon snack:** mango and papaya smoothie (see page 153) or fresh fruit **Dinner:** Cuban chicken (see page 147). Brown rice. Hot bananas with pumpkin seeds & lime (see page 150) **Drinks:** 2½ cups 1% or 2% milk. Unsweetened fresh fruit juice. Unlimited green, black, white, or herbal tea, and mineral water. 5 ounces (⅔ cup) red wine or unsweetened red grape juice **Supplements:** see page 116

DAILY EXERCISE ROUTINE

Start with the head/neck stretch from day one and follow it with this shoulder-loosening exercise. Also walk briskly for 15 to 20 minutes during the day.

SHOULDER LOOSENING

1 Stand comfortably, with your feet apart. Clasp your hands behind your head.
2 Pull your elbows forward so they almost touch in front of your face. Then move your elbows out until they are as wide apart as possible.

GRAPEFRUIT—EAT WITH CAUTION

Before you eat grapefruit, read the drug information sheet that comes with any medication you take. Grapefruit affects the absorption of some drugs, including statins and the calcium channel blocker class of anti-hypertensive drugs. This effect can be large. For example, taking one particular statin drug (lovastatin) with a glass of grapefruit juice produces the same blood levels of the drug as taking 12 tablets. If necessary, replace grapefruit with an orange—a blood orange if they are in season.

3 Repeat several times until your shoulders have loosened up.

AROMATHERAPY

Have a blood pressure-lowering bath before bed. Add the following essential oils to 15 ml of carrier oil (see page 39): 1 drop lavender, 2 drops geranium, 3 drops marjoram. Add the mixture to a warm bath, light some candles, and soak for 15 minutes with your eyes closed. Before getting out, use a sponge to collect oil from the surface of the water and then massage onto your skin. Place lavender oil under your pillow again.

DAY THREE

DAILY MENU

Breakfast: Bircher muesli (see page 142) with a handful of mixed berries
Morning snack: a piece of fruit
Lunch: carrot and cilantro soup (see page 143). Wholewheat roll. Bowl of mixed salad leaves. Low-fat yogurt with live cultures with fresh fruit
Afternoon snack: a handful of walnuts or a piece of fresh fruit
Dinner: sliced tomato sprinkled with torn basil and olive oil. Trout with almonds and sweet potatoes (see page 149). Spinach. Corn kernels

Drinks: 2½ cups 1% or 2% milk. Unsweetened fresh fruit juice. Unlimited green, black, white, or herbal tea, and mineral water. 5 ounces (⅔ cup) red wine or unsweetened red grape juice
Supplements: see page 116

DAILY EXERCISE ROUTINE

Do the exercises from days one and two, and then add the following exercise, which mobilizes and stretches your upper body and helps to promote flexibility in your spine. For cardiovascular exercise, walk briskly for 15 to 20 minutes today.

SIDE STRETCH

1 Stand with your feet roughly shoulder-width apart. Slowly raise your arms above your head. Let your spine become long.

2 Bring your fingertips together above your head. Keep your neck and shoulders relaxed.

3 Slowly lean to the right with your upper body. Feel the stretch along your left side. Now stretch to the left.

AROMATHERAPY

Camomile essential oil has soothing, calming properties. Put a few drops of camomile German or camomile Roman essential oil on cotton ball and place it in a small plastic box with a tightly fitting lid.

Open the box and inhale the scent deeply at intervals throughout the day. Continue to use lavender essential oil under your pillow when you go to bed.

TASTY SALADS

To add extra flavor to today's lunchtime mixed leaf salad, sprinkle freshly chopped herbs and a little crushed garlic on the leaves. You can make a delicious dressing by combining 2 tbsp. walnut oil with the juice of one lemon or lime in a screw-top jar and shaking. Walnut oil is a good source of omega-3 fatty acids, which have a thinning action on blood that helps lower blood pressure. You can additionally increase the omega-3 content of a salad by sprinkling it with nuts and seeds.

DAY FOUR

DAILY MENU

Breakfast: homemade smoothie—whiz together one small banana with ⅔ cup plain low-fat yogurt with live cultures, plus a handful of almonds
Morning snack: a piece of fruit
Lunch: broiled tomatoes with spinach on rye (see page 143). Bowl of mixed salad leaves drizzled with walnut oil. Low-fat yogurt with live cultures with black grapes
Afternoon snack: a handful of mixed nuts
Dinner: warm Mediterranean vegetable salad with balsamic dressing (see page 149). Wholewheat pasta. Bowl of mixed salad leaves. Baked peaches with raspberries (see page 151)
Drinks: 2½ cups 1% or 2% milk. Unsweetened fresh fruit juice. Unlimited green, black, white, or herbal tea, and mineral water. 5 ounces (⅔ cup) red wine or unsweetened red grape juice
Supplements: see page 116

Having something for breakfast is very important, even if it's just a smoothie, as in today's breakfast. Researchers from Harvard Medical School have found that people who eat breakfast are 30 percent less likely to be obese than those who skip this important first meal of the day.

DAILY EXERCISE ROUTINE

Do the exercises from days one to three, and then add the following exercise. Also walk briskly for 15 to 20 minutes.

FORWARD ARM STRETCH

1 Extend your arms in front of you at shoulder height.
2 Interlink your fingers and turn your palms outward.

FLUID INTAKE

Lack of fluids can increase blood stickiness and might promote formation of abnormal blood clots. Don't wait until you are thirsty to drink—this is a sign of dehydration.

3 Stretch your hands forward as far as you can and hold for 10 seconds.

4 Relax, then repeat. Release your arms.

AROMATHERAPY

Make up a new camomile essential oil inhaling box and inhale regularly throughout the day. In addition, start drinking camomile tea for its relaxing properties. Camomile teabags are available in supermarkets and whole-food stores. Continue to use lavender essential oil at night.

DAY FIVE

DAILY MENU

Breakfast: homemade muesli (see page 141)
Morning snack: a piece of fruit
Lunch: corn-on-the-cob. Bowl of mixed salad leaves drizzled with walnut oil. Wholewheat roll. Low-fat yogurt with live cultures with fresh fruit

Afternoon snack: a handful of grapes (preferably black or red)
Dinner: bulgur wheat with peppers and bean sprouts (see page 148). Broiled chicken breast or salmon steak. Green vegetables, such as broccoli, bok choy, or green beans. Low-fat

fromage blanc with fresh fruit
Drinks: 2½ cups 1% or 2% milk. Unsweetened fresh fruit juice. Unlimited green, black, white, or herbal tea, and mineral water. 5 ounces (⅔ cup) red wine or unsweetened red grape juice
Supplements: see page 116

DAILY EXERCISE ROUTINE

Do the exercises from days one through four, and then add the following exercise. Also walk briskly for 15 to 20 minutes.

WAIST TWISTS

1 Stand comfortably with your feet apart and your hands on your hips.

2 Without moving your lower body, rotate your upper body and hips to the right, as far as you can and back again. Then rotate as far as you can to the left, then back. Repeat five times on each side.

DRINKING LESS ALCOHOL

If you drank a lot of alcohol before starting this program and are finding it difficult to cut back, you might find a supplement called kudzu (*Pueraria lobata*; see page 48) helps.

AROMATHERAPY

If you spend most of the day working alone, use an essential oil burner to scent the room with a blend of anti-hypertensive essential oils. Using two or more complementary essential oils together has a synergistic effect that is more powerful than using each on their own. Use 5 drops each of marjoram, lavender, and clary sage. Alternatively, add the drops to a cotton ball placed in a small plastic box you can open and inhale regularly during the day—inhale deeply and then make your exhalation long and slow until your lungs feel empty. Breathe in and out like this two or three times. This is a good technique to use when you're feeling very stressed. Continue to use lavender essential oil to help you sleep.

DAY SIX

DAILY MENU

Breakfast: banana-cinnamon oatmeal (see page 141)
Morning snack: a piece of fruit
Lunch: Waldorf salad with red pepper (see page 145). Bowl of mixed salad leaves drizzled with walnut oil. Low-fat yogurt with live cultures with fresh fruit
Afternoon snack: a handful of almonds
Dinner: salmon with red pepper sauté (see page 146). Spinach. Wholewheat pasta. About 1½ ounces dark chocolate

Drinks: 2½ cups 1% or 2% milk. Unsweetened fresh fruit juice. Unlimited green, black, white, or herbal tea, and mineral water. 5 ounces (²⁄₃ cup) red wine or unsweetened red grape juice
Supplements: see page 116

Eating oats in the form of oatmeal (or muesli) for breakfast can help to lower your blood pressure. Recent research shows the daily consumption of whole oats can lower blood pressure by 7.5/5.5 mmHg over six weeks (compared with no change in those not eating oatmeal).

Researchers concluded the soluble fiber in oatmeal is an effective dietary therapy in both the prevention and treatment of hypertension. I suggest you include oats in your future long-term diet as frequently as possible.

DAILY EXERCISE ROUTINE

Do the exercises from days one through five, and then add the following exercise. Start increasing the distance you walk: spend 20 to 25 minutes on brisk walking today.

FORWARD BENDS

1 Stand comfortably with your feet apart.
2 Let your body curl slowly forward from your waist, keeping your legs straight, until your hands are as close to the floor as possible.
3 Touch the floor if you can.
4 Slowly straighten up. Repeat four times.

AROMATHERAPY

When you use the same aromatherapy oil regularly, it becomes less effective as your body adapts to its therapeutic action. So, instead of lavender oil to promote sleep, start using 2 drops each of lemongrass and orange essential oils near your pillow at night for the next five nights.

From now on, I recommend you change your nightly essential oil at least once a week.

FISH OIL AND GARLIC

Whenever you eat oily fish, such as salmon, I recommend adding plenty of garlic to the accompanying marinade or dressing. Fish oil and garlic have a synergistic effect. Research shows that daily garlic supplements and fish oil supplements can reduce LDL-cholesterol by 20 percent and triglycerides by 37 percent within two months. This has a blood-thinning effect that reduces hypertension.

DAY SEVEN

DAILY MENU

Breakfast: broiled tomatoes on toast sprinkled with arugula and olive oil
Morning snack: a piece of fruit
Lunch: guacamole (see page 152). Wholewheat toast, rice cakes, or crispbread. Bowl of mixed salad leaves drizzled with walnut oil. Low-fat yogurt with live cultures with fresh fruit
Afternoon snack: a handful of almonds
Dinner: lamb shanks in red wine (see page 150). Green leafy vegetable, such as broccoli or spinach. Wholewheat pasta. Poire au chocolat (see page 151)
Drinks: 2½ cups 1% or 2% milk. Unsweetened fresh fruit juice. Unlimited green, black, white, or herbal tea, and mineral water. 5 ounces (²⁄₃ cup) red wine or unsweetened red grape juice
Supplements: see page 116

Before you broil your tomatoes for breakfast today, drizzle them with olive oil. Cooking tomatoes in olive oil releases the most lycopene for absorption. Lycopene is an antioxidant found in tomatoes that can help lower blood pressure. The lycopene content of tomatoes is relatively small; red varieties contain the most and yellow varieties the least. The best and most concentrated source is a supplement.

DAILY EXERCISE ROUTINE
Do the exercises from days one through six, and then add the following exercise. Continue to walk briskly for 20 to 25 minutes today.

THIGH STRETCHES
1 Stand comfortably, feet apart, with the back of a chair to your left. Keep your back and head straight, and your abdomen and pelvis tucked in.
2 Rest your left hand on the back of the chair for support. Bend your left knee slightly for support, then lift your right foot until you can grasp your right ankle behind you with your right hand. Keep your knees facing forward.
3 Gently ease your foot in toward your bottom until you feel a mild stretch in your thigh.

4 Hold for a count of five. Turn round and repeat the stretch on your left leg.

CONSULTING A HOMEOPATH

Having followed the gentle program for one week, your blood pressure should already have reduced, especially if you're taking the supplements on page 116. You might now like to consult a therapist; I suggest you start with a course of homeopathy. To find a homeopath, check the resources on page 237. A homeopath selects remedies based on your symptoms and constitutional type (of which there are 15). He or she determines your constitutional type according to your body shape, demeanor, and personality. This involves answering questions about your likes, dislikes, fears, food preferences, and emotions. Prescribing according to your constitutional type is important when treating a long-term condition, such as hypertension, because each constitutional type has its own remedies that will work best.

DAY EIGHT

DAILY MENU

Breakfast: low-fat yogurt with live cultures with fresh berries
Morning snack: a piece of fruit
Lunch: bowl of home-made coleslaw (toss finely shredded cabbage, onion, and carrot in low-fat mayonnaise). Bowl of mixed salad leaves drizzled with walnut oil. Wholewheat roll. Low-fat fromage blanc with fruit
Afternoon snack: a handful of mixed nuts
Dinner: garlic chicken (see page 145). Carrots. Spring greens. Unsweetened summer pudding (see page 152)
Drinks: 2½ cups 1% or 2% milk. Unsweetened fresh fruit juice. Unlimited green, black, white, or herbal tea, and mineral water. 5 ounces (⅔ cup) red wine or unsweetened red grape juice
Supplements: see page 116

DAILY EXERCISE ROUTINE

Over the next week, I introduce some simple yoga poses that will help you to relax physically and mentally at the end of the day. The first is

A VEGETARIAN DIET
People who follow a vegetarian diet tend to have a systolic blood pressure that is around 5 mmHg lower than meat eaters. This reduction occurs within six weeks of omitting meat from the diet (and blood pressure rises to its previous levels within six weeks of eating meat again).

mountain pose, which helps improve your body alignment. Continue your morning exercises (see days one through seven) and your 20 to 25-minute brisk walk.

MOUNTAIN POSE
1 Stand with your feet slightly apart, toes facing forward.
2 Keep your back straight and your arms by your sides, with your palms facing inward.
3 Spread your toes and roll your pelvis forward slightly so your tailbone tucks under.
4 Pull in your tummy muscles. Tighten your pelvic floor muscles.
5 As you inhale, roll your shoulders back and down, so your chest moves forward a little.
6 Press your feet down firmly into the floor. Imagine someone is holding your hair and pulling you up from your crown.
7 Relax your upper body. Breathe in and out slowly and deeply 10 times.

MEDITATION
Over the next week I explain several ways of meditating that will help you switch off your body's reaction to stress. For your first meditation, sit in a chair with your eyes shut. Imagine your favorite color. Some people visualize color as a dot; others as a moving cloud; others as a wash of even color. In general, the more color you visualize, the stronger the therapeutic effect. Focus on and explore your chosen color. If your mind wanders, bring it back to the color. When you feel ready, bring your mind back, open your eyes, and enjoy a sense of calm.

DAY NINE

DAILY MENU

Breakfast: Bircher muesli (see page 142)
Morning snack: a piece of fruit
Lunch: carrot and cilantro soup (see page 143). Bowl of mixed salad leaves drizzled with walnut oil. Low-fat cottage cheese.

Wholewheat roll. Low-fat yogurt with live cultures with fresh fruit
Afternoon snack: a handful of brazil nuts
Dinner: Mexican spiced turkey (see page 147). Brown rice. Fresh figs
Drinks: 2½ cups 1% or 2%

milk. Unsweetened fresh fruit juice. Unlimited green, black, white, or herbal tea, and mineral water. 5 ounces (⅔ cup) red wine or unsweetened red grape juice
Supplements: see page 116

Today's dinnertime dessert is figs. Figs are an excellent source of potassium, which helps to reduce blood pressure by flushing excess sodium and fluids from the body via your kidneys. Figs are also one of the richest dietary sources of soluble fiber and help reduce cholesterol and triglyceride levels (see pages 72–73). They are delicious eaten fresh. You can also freeze fresh figs—because they don't freeze hard, you can eat them straight from the freezer as a snack.

DAILY EXERCISE ROUTINE

Do the first yoga pose in your evening sequence (see day eight), and then do the following leg stretch. Continue to do your morning exercises (see days one through seven) and your daily 20 to 25-minute walk.

WIDE-LEG STRETCH

1 From the mountain pose, inhale deeply then move your feet wide apart and point your toes comfortably inward. Put your hands on your hips

WHEN TO AVOID BRISK EXERCISE

You should avoid brisk exercise for two hours after eating a meal, and late in the evening as it can keep you awake. A gentle stroll before sleep is fine, however.

and, as you slowly breathe out, bend forward from your hips, keeping your spine straight.

2 Keep your legs straight, push down through your feet and lift your tailbone. Keep your chest facing forward.

3 Try to lengthen your spine as much as possible. Hold the stretch for five slow, deep breaths.

MEDITATION

Today, weather permitting, I'd like you to sit in a shady, private spot outdoors, perhaps in your garden or a park. Close your eyes and immerse yourself in the relaxing qualities of nature for 10 to 20 minutes. Try to isolate all the different sounds you can hear—insects buzzing, birds singing, wind rustling in the trees. Notice the way the light intensity on your eyelids varies with the dappling effects of leaves and moving clouds. Focus on the breeze caressing your skin, or the sun's warmth. Smell the damp, earthy or warm herby odors around you. If thoughts of life and work intrude, gently bring your awareness back to your contemplation of your surroundings. When you're ready, stand up, breathe in deeply and stretch. Now enjoy your day.

DAY TEN

DAILY MENU

Breakfast: homemade muesli (see page 141). Low-fat yogurt
Morning snack: a piece of fruit
Lunch: smoked trout and lemon pâté (see page 153). Wholewheat toast or oatcakes. Arugula. Low-fat yogurt with live cultures with mango cubes

Afternoon snack: a handful of mixed nuts
Dinner: Cuban chicken (see page 147). Roast baby vine tomatoes. Bowl of mixed salad leaves drizzled with walnut oil. Hot bananas with pumpkin seeds and lime

(see page 150)
Drinks: 2½ cups 1% or 2% milk. Unsweetened fresh fruit juice. Unlimited green, black, white, or herbal tea, and mineral water. 5 ounces (⅔ cup) red wine or unsweetened red grape juice
Supplements: see page 116

DAILY EXERCISE ROUTINE

Do the first two yoga poses in your evening sequence (see days eight and nine), and then add the following pose. Continue to do your morning exercises (see days one through seven), and your daily 20 to 25-minute walk.

DOWNWARD DOG

1 Start on all fours with your knees together and your hands firmly on the floor, shoulder-width apart.
2 Lift your knees off the ground and push your tailbone high in the air so your body makes a wide inverted "V" shape. Your arms and legs should be straight.
3 Pull your tummy in toward your spine and lift your pelvic floor muscles. Press your heels and the palms of your hands into the floor. Don't let them slide away. Let your spine become long. Hold this posture for five slow, deep breaths, then relax.

MEDITATION

Yesterday, you sat in quiet contemplation with nature. Today, I'd like you to sit quietly and focus on your body. Breathe in and out slowly and deeply. Be mindful of what happens when you breathe. Follow the passage of air through your nostrils or lips. Observe how your abdomen rises as you inhale, and falls as you exhale, and how your ribcage expands to pull air into your body, then contracts to push air out. Note whether your breath is shallow or deep, smooth or ragged. Focus on your circulation. Become aware of your heart beating and blood pulsing through your arteries.

The more you focus on your body, the more you switch off from the world. Do this for 15 minutes, or as long as you like.

EAT MORE CARROTS
Carrots contain substances called cumarin glycosides that reduce arterial blood pressure through actions similar to that of calcium channel blockers (see page 24).

DAY ELEVEN

DAILY MENU

Breakfast: frittata (see page 142). Arugula. Wholewheat toast
Morning snack: orange and carrot juice (see page 152)
Lunch: tuna, bean, and pepper salad (see page 144). Wholewheat roll.

Low-fat yogurt with live cultures with fresh fruit
Afternoon snack: a handful of mixed nuts
Dinner: halibut with tarragon sauce (see page 148). Corn kernels. Spinach. A handful of red or black grapes

Drinks: 2½ cups 1% or 2% milk. Unsweetened fresh fruit juice. Unlimited green, black, white, or herbal tea, and mineral water. 5 ounces (⅔ cup) red wine or unsweetened red grape juice
Supplements: see page 116

Make today's breakfast with omega-3 enriched eggs. Research shows that eating four enriched eggs a week for four weeks not only significantly reduces your systolic blood pressure, it also lowers your triglyceride level (and does not raise your cholesterol levels).

DAILY EXERCISE ROUTINE

Do the first three yoga poses in your evening sequence (see days eight through ten), and then add the following pose. Continue to do your morning exercises (see days one through seven) and your daily 20 to 25-minute brisk walk.

THE PLANK

1 From downward dog (see day ten) lower your bottom so your legs, back, and head form a straight line—like a plank.
2 Gently tuck your chin in and look at the floor. Let your weight rest on your toes and palms (spread your fingers and thumbs). Pull your tummy in toward your spine and squeeze your pelvic floor muscles.
3 Maintain this pose for five slow, deep breaths.

MEDITATION

By focusing your mind on a particular object, such as a mandala, you can screen out distractions and, with time and practice, you can enter a state of profound relaxation and serenity. A mandala is a diagram whose name derives from the Sanskrit word for "circle."

Today, I'd like you to find a mandala and spend 15 minutes focusing on it. You can search for mandalas on the internet or create your own using colours and shapes that please you—look in books or online for inspiration. (You can also gaze at the patterns in a child's kaleidoscope.) During your contemplation, let your gaze wander over the shapes and angles of the mandala. Absorb the colors and patterns into your mind.

DAY TWELVE

DAILY MENU

Breakfast: homemade muesli (see page 141) with kiwi

Morning snack: a piece of fruit

Lunch: carrot and cilantro soup (see page 143). Wholewheat roll. Bowl of mixed salad leaves drizzled with walnut oil.

Low-fat yogurt with live cultures with fresh fruit

Afternoon snack: a handful of mixed nuts

Dinner: smoked mackerel mixed with mango cubes and piled onto mixed salad leaves. About 1½ ounces dark chocolate

Drinks: 2½ cups 1% or 2% milk. Unsweetened fresh fruit juice. Unlimited green, black, white, or herbal tea, and mineral water. 5 ounces (⅔ cup) red wine or unsweetened red grape juice

Supplements: see page 116

The mackerel in today's lunch is a rich source of omega-3 fatty acids; it provides twice as much as herring. Mackerel is also special in that it reduces renin activity (see page 16) by more than 60 percent. So, when buying oily fish, make mackerel your first choice.

DAILY EXERCISE ROUTINE

Do the first four yoga poses in your evening sequence (see days eight through eleven), and then add the following pose. Continue to do your morning exercises (see days one through seven) and, from today, increase your daily walk to 25 to 30 minutes.

FOUR-LIMB STAFF POSE

1 From plank pose (see page 132), slowly bend your arms and lower your body until it's close to the floor. Squeeze your elbows in to your ribcage. Pull your tummy toward your spine, lift your pelvic floor muscles, and tuck in your chin. Lengthen your spine.

2 Hover a little way off the floor with only your toes and hands in contact with the ground. Hold this sticklike posture for five slow, deep breaths.

MEDITATION

Select an aromatherapy candle with a relaxing scent, such as lavender, geranium or lemongrass. (For more about the qualities of different essential oils, see page 42.) Sit in a quiet room, on the floor or at a table. Light the candle and place it on a plate a short distance away from you.

Focus on the flame. Look deeply into it. Explore it and watch how it flickers in front of you. As thoughts enter your head, notice them and then just quietly let them go again. Keep returning your attention to the flame. After a while, close your eyes and watch the flame dance in your mind's eye. If the image starts to fade, just open your eyes to look at the flame again. Do this meditation for up to 20 minutes before safely extinguishing the flame.

DAY THIRTEEN

DAILY MENU

Breakfast: fresh fruit smoothie (see day four). Wholewheat toast
Morning snack: a piece of fruit
Lunch: pear, avocado, and nut salad (see page 145). Bowl of mixed salad leaves drizzled with walnut oil. Low-fat yogurt

with live cultures with fresh fruit
Afternoon snack: smoked trout and lemon pâté (see page 153)
Dinner: slice of melon. Bulgur wheat with peppers and bean sprouts (see page 148). Broiled chicken or salmon steak

Drinks: 2½ cups 1% or 2% milk. Unsweetened fresh fruit juice. Unlimited green, black, white, or herbal tea, and mineral water. 5 ounces (⅔ cup) red wine or unsweetened red grape juice
Supplements: see page 116

You should be in the habit of eating yogurt with live cultures every day by now. This yogurt contains probiotic bacteria that break down milk proteins. During this process, peptides are produced, which have anti-hypertensive properties.

DAILY EXERCISE ROUTINE
Do the first five yoga poses in your evening sequence (see days eight through twelve), and then add the cobra. Continue to do your morning exercises (see days one through seven) and walk for 25 to 30 minutes.

THE COBRA
1 From the four-limb staff pose, let your body drop gently to the floor.
2 Let your legs relax and your toes point out behind you.
3 With your hands just under your shoulders, lift your head, neck, and upper chest, keeping your head in line with your spine. Keep your hips on the floor and your legs relaxed.
4 Look forward and up while supporting your weight on your palms. Maintain this posture for five slow, deep breaths.

CRYSTAL MEDITATION
Crystals can greatly enhance the power of a meditation. Select a crystal you feel particularly drawn to, or choose from those traditionally used to reduce blood pressure and induce relaxation: amethyst (calming and relaxing); aventurine (increases creativity and reduces hypertension); sodalite (boosts endurance and helps to reduce hypertension); or prehnite (used where hypertension is associated with kidney problems).

Sit comfortably in a quiet room and hold your chosen crystal in your hands. Close your eyes and try to picture the crystal in your mind's eye. Let the colors, shapes, and textures of the crystal swirl through your mind, as it draws you deeper down into a quiet, relaxing space.

If your mind wanders, open your eyes and gaze at the crystal's shape. It is surprisingly easy to imagine yourself inside the crystal exploring its many facets. In your own time, bring the meditation to a close—about 20 minutes is a good length of time to spend on this relaxing therapy.

DAY FOURTEEN

DAILY MENU

Breakfast: banana-cinnamon oatmeal (see page 141)
Morning snack: a piece of fruit
Lunch: coronation turkey salad with cranberries (see page 144). Bowl of mixed salad leaves drizzled with walnut oil. Wholewheat roll. Low-fat yogurt with live cultures with fresh fruit
Afternoon snack: fruit smoothie
Dinner: half an avocado sprinkled with chopped walnuts. Baked oriental salmon (see page 146). Broccoli. Carrots
Drinks: 2½ cups 1% or 2% milk. Unsweetened fresh fruit juice. Unlimited green, black, white, or herbal tea, and mineral water. 5 ounces (⅔ cup) red wine or unsweetened red grape juice
Supplements: see page 116

DAILY EXERCISE ROUTINE

Do the first six yoga poses in your evening sequence (see days eight through thirteen), and then add the corpse pose. Continue to do your morning exercises (see days one through seven) and walk for 25 to 30 minutes. From now on, try to walk briskly for at least 30 minutes on most days of the week. To add variety to your cardiovascular exercise routine, try replacing walking with swimming, dancing, or cycling on some days.

THE CORPSE POSE

1 Lie on your back with your arms out to the sides and your palms facing upward. Start with your feet pointing up, then let your hips rotate so your feet drop comfortably out to either side.

2 Close your eyes and allow every muscle in your body to relax as if you are sinking into the floor. Mentally scan your body for any remaining pockets of tension.

3 Breathe slowly and softly, and try to feel the flow of energy through your body. Stay in this posture for 5 to 10 minutes.

CONSULTING AN AROMATHERAPIST

Now you are at the end of the program, I suggest you try a relaxing and therapeutic aromatherapy massage. To find an aromatherapist, check the resources at the end of this book (see page 237). An aromatherapist will select essential oils that help to lower blood pressure and encourage you to relax. During your first session, he or she will ask questions about your medical history and lifestyle. The therapist might select the oils themselves or invite you to choose your preferred aromas from a selection. Aromatherapy massage is usually based on Swedish massage techniques and can also involve acupressure. A full-body massage lasts about 60 minutes. You will feel relaxed and, often, sleepy afterward. An aromatherapist might supply oils for you to take home and inhale or massage into your skin. A medical aromatherapist might also prescribe aromatherapy oils for internal use—never consume aromatherapy oils except under professional supervision. If you enjoy the massage, book yourself in for four weekly sessions.

CONTINUING THE GENTLE PROGRAM

You have now followed the gentle program for two weeks —congratulations! I suggest you continue with the eating plan for another two weeks. This way you will have a month of healthy eating behind you, and you will be very familiar with the foods you need to shop for and eat every day. You can vary the foods you eat, and include some new recipes. You will find some new recipe suggestions at www.naturalhealthguru.co.uk. You can also post your own favorites there for other followers of the plan to try. The information below will help you map out your future using the principles of the gentle program.

YOUR LONG-TERM DIET
The gentle program provides a simple diet based on healthy, low-glycemic principles such as those described in the DASH diet (see page 66). This encourages you to eat plenty of whole grains, fruits, vegetables, low-fat dairy products, fish, poultry, nuts, and beans, while cutting back on red meat, candy, saturated fats, and sodium. Continue to eat according to

these principles. This checklist enables you to see at a glance what healthy adults should be eating each day:

- At least 2½ cups fruit and 2½ cups vegetables every day.
- At least 6 ounces of whole grains. A 1-ounce serving is equivalent to one slice wholegrain bread or 1 cup ready-to-eat cereal, or ½ cup of cooked rice or wholewheat pasta.
- No more than 5 to 6½ ounces a day, depending on your age and gender, of lean meats, poultry, eggs, fish, legumes, nuts, and seeds. Select omega-3 enriched hen's eggs whenever possible as, unlike normal hen's eggs, these have beneficial effects on your blood pressure and blood cholesterol levels.

ADAPTING RECIPES

You can usually adapt recipes from any cookbook to meet the principles of the gentle program. Here are some guidelines:

- Omit salt or sugar from recipes. You can add honey occasionally if additional sweetness is desirable.
- Make food tasty by adding lots of freshly chopped herbs. If you have space in your garden or on your windowsill to grow herbs, this can become a rewarding hobby.
- Replace light cream with low-fat plain yogurt and heavy cream with fromage blanc. Experiment to see what works best.
- Add yogurt to sauces or casseroles off the heat, and don't add yogurt to liquids at boiling point—the mixture can curdle. This won't affect the flavor, but it looks unsightly.
- You can make yogurt less likely to curdle by stabilizing it. Stir in one teaspoon cornstarch ⅔ cup yogurt before using it in a recipe.
- Rather than using yogurt as a topping for baked dishes, use fromage blanc (yogurt protein coagulates). Alternatively, add yogurt (mixed with herbs and seasoning) after the dish is out of the oven.

BURN OFF CALORIES BY WALKING

Exercise can burn a surprising number of calories and will help to keep your weight down, as well as your blood pressure. For example, walking briskly (4½ miles per hour) for 30 minutes burns 200 calories. Walking is an ideal form of exercise if you have previously been inactive for a long time. You can start very gently and build up the intensity as your fitness levels improve.

YOUR LONG-TERM SUPPLEMENT REGIME

Continue taking the recommended supplements for the gentle program (see page 116) long term. Research supports their use at this level for gentle yet significant effects on your blood pressure and future health. If, until now, you have taken only the supplements in the recommended list, you might wish to add in one or more of the supplements in the optional list for additional benefits.

Go to pages 86–92 to find more information about the supplements in which you are interested.

YOUR EXERCISE ROUTINE

After just two weeks of regular exercise you should have started to notice a difference in your fitness level. Continue with your morning exercise regime at the beginning of the day. Fit in at least 30 minutes of brisk exercise during the day. This can be walking, cycling, swimming, dancing, or gardening—whatever activity you enjoy and can fit into your lifestyle. Vary the type of exercise you do from day to day. Then, at the end of each day, do the wind-down yoga sequence to lower your blood pressure and relax you in preparation for a good night's sleep.

YOUR THERAPY PROGRAM

The gentle program has shown you how to use aromatherapy techniques and meditation for relaxation. Although these activities might seem simple, don't underestimate the powerful effect they can have on your cardiovascular health and general well-being. Try to practise one meditation technique each day—or combine the two therapies by meditating while scenting the room with your favorite essential oils. If you found the homeopathy and aromatherapy appointments useful, continue to go to sessions on a regular basis.

MONITORING YOUR BLOOD PRESSURE

I suggest you monitor your blood pressure on a weekly basis, at the same time of day each time, unless your doctor has asked you to check it more frequently. Record your blood pressure measurements in a chart, such as the one on page 112. This will give you an instant visual indication of whether your blood pressure is going down (as it should during this program), staying the same, or going up.

If your blood pressure is consistently below 130/80 mmHg, well done—this program has worked well for you. You might now want to discuss with your doctor the ways in which your treatment can change to reflect your lower blood pressure. It's important to be aware, however, that the dose of some anti-hypertensive drugs must be reduced slowly to prevent any rebound effects in which your blood pressure quickly bounces back up again.

If your blood pressure is consistently between 130/80 mmHg and 140/90 mmHg, consider moving up to the moderate program (see pages 154–196) to see if you can bring it down to below 130/80 mmHg.

If your blood pressure is consistently above 140/90 mmHg, move onto the moderate program, but consult your doctor for individual advice.

BREAKFAST RECIPES

HOMEMADE MUESLI

SERVES 4

1 handful oatmeal
3 handfuls mixed cereals (toasted wheat, rye, barley, and bran flakes)
1 handful mixed nuts, such as walnuts, Brazil nuts, and slivered almonds, roughly chopped
1 handful mixed seeds, such as sunflower, pumpkin, and sesame seeds
1 handful raisins or golden raisins
1 handful chopped apricots, dates, or figs (optional)
Milk, to serve

1 Mix together all the ingredients except the milk in a large bowl.

2 Divide between four serving bowls and pour over enough milk to taste.

BANANA-CINNAMON OATMEAL

SERVES 4

2½ cups water
1½ cups unsweetened instant oatmeal
1 teaspoon freshly ground cinnamon
1 large banana, sliced

1 Bring the water to boiling point in a medium saucepan. Add the oatmeal and a good sprinkling of the cinnamon. Simmer gently, stirring continuously, about 1 minute. Remove from the heat, cover, and leave at least 5 minutes, until all the liquid is absorbed.

2 Divide between four serving bowls and top with the banana and the remaining cinnamon.

BIRCHER MUESLI

SERVES 4

1 sweet apple
Grated peel and freshly squeezed juice
   of 1 unwaxed lemon
2 cups oatmeal
2½ cups low-fat soy or almond milk (or
   low-fat yogurt with live cultures)
⅔ cup raisins
1 banana, thinly sliced
1 orange, peeled and roughly chopped
1 handful chopped nuts
1 handful fresh seasonal fruit, such as
   berries, peaches, nectarines, pears,
   or cherries, roughly chopped if
   necessary, to serve

1 Peel and core the apple. Grate into
   a bowl, then sprinkle the lemon juice
   and peel over (to prevent the apple
   discoloring).

2 Add the oatmeal, milk, raisins,
   banana, and orange flesh and mix
   well. Cover and leave in the
   refrigerator overnight.

3 Divide between four serving bowls.
   Serve with a topping of chopped nuts
   and fresh seasonal fruit.

FRITTATA

SERVES 4

8 organic omega-3 enriched eggs
½ tablespoon olive oil
2 shallots, sliced
2 garlic cloves, crushed
1 red or orange bell pepper, sliced
3 large handfuls fresh spinach, washed
   and roughly chopped
4 tomatoes, sliced
1 handful fresh basil leaves, torn
Freshly ground black pepper
1 small bunch watercress, to serve

1 Heat the broiler to hot. Beat the eggs
   well and season to taste with black
   pepper. Set aside.

2 Heat a nonstick skillet until hot. Add
   the oil, then the shallots, garlic, and
   red pepper and sauté over medium
   heat 5 minutes. Pour the egg mixture
   over, followed by the spinach,
   tomatoes, and basil. Cook over low
   heat, without stirring, 3 minutes.

3 Put the pan under the hot broiler and
   leave until the top of the frittata is
   golden brown. Serve, garnished with
   sprigs of watercress.

LUNCH RECIPES

CARROT AND CILANTRO SOUP

SERVES 4

1½ teaspoons olive oil
1 onion, finely chopped
2 garlic cloves, crushed
4 cups grated or finely chopped carrots, plus 1 carrot, grated, to serve
1 tablespoon coriander seeds, crushed or ground
3 cups vegetable stock (see page 153) or water
Freshly squeezed lemon juice, to taste
6 tablespoons low-fat yogurt with live cultures
1 handful fresh cilantro leaves, roughly chopped
Pinch of nutmeg, grated (optional)
Freshly ground black pepper

1 Heat the oil in a large pan. Add the onion and garlic and fry slowly until soft.

2 Add the carrots, coriander seeds, and stock and bring to a boil. Reduce the heat and simmer 20 minutes. Leave to cool a little, then purée in a blender. Season with black pepper and lemon juice.

3 Return to the pan and heat gently. Serve topped with yogurt, grated carrot, chopped cilantro, and nutmeg, if using.

BROILED TOMATOES WITH SPINACH ON RYE

SERVES 4

4 large slices rye bread
Extra virgin olive oil or walnut oil, for drizzling
3 large handfuls spinach leaves, washed and wilted in a steamer
4 ripe medium tomatoes, thinly sliced
4 thin slices mozzarella cheese (optional)
Freshly ground black pepper

1 Heat the broiler to hot, then lightly toast the rye bread on both sides.

2 Remove from the broiler and drizzle a little oil over each piece of toast. Arrange the spinach and tomatoes on top. Drizzle a little more oil over or, if preferred, top with mozzarella cheese. Season to taste with black pepper.

3 Return to the hot broiler for a few minutes, until lightly brown or the cheese melts. Serve immediately.

TUNA, BEAN AND PEPPER SALAD

SERVES 4

1 can (15-oz.) mixed beans, drained
1 can (7-oz.) tuna in spring water or olive oil (not brine), drained
1 red bell pepper, seeded and chopped
1 green bell pepper, seeded and chopped
1 red onion, finely chopped
1 handful fresh flat-leaf parsley, finely chopped

For the dressing:
2 tablespoons extra virgin olive oil or walnut oil
2 tablespoons red wine vinegar
1 garlic clove, crushed
Freshly ground black pepper

1 Mix the beans, tuna, peppers, red onion, and parsley together in a bowl.

2 To make the dressing, put the oil, vinegar, and garlic in a screw-top jar; shake and season with black pepper. Pour the dressing over the salad and toss well.

CORONATION TURKEY SALAD WITH CRANBERRIES

SERVES 4

1 large handful dried cranberries
4 tablespoons red wine vinegar
1½ tablespoons olive oil
1 tablespoon curry powder
1 iceberg lettuce, shredded
⅔ cup low-fat yogurt with live cultures or fromage blanc
4 cups cooked, cubed turkey breast
1 carrot, grated
1 cucumber, seeded and finely chopped
1 handful fresh cilantro leaves, finely chopped
3 tablespoons slivered almonds
Freshly ground black pepper

1 Microwave the dried cranberries and vinegar on a high setting for 90 seconds.

2 Heat the oil in a pan. Add the curry powder and stir-fry 1 minute. Add the cranberries and vinegar and stir-fry 1 minute longer. Transfer to a large bowl and put in the refrigerator about 5 minutes. Put the lettuce in a large serving bowl.

3 Mix the yogurt with the cool cranberry mixture and season with black pepper. Fold in the turkey, carrot, cucumber, and cilantro leaves. Pile on top of the lettuce. Sprinkle the slivered almonds over and serve.

DINNER RECIPES

WALDORF SALAD WITH RED PEPPER

SERVES 4

4 red apples, peeled, cored, and chopped
Grated peel and freshly squeezed juice
   of 1 unwaxed lemon
⅔ cup low-fat fromage blanc
4 celery stalks, chopped
1 red bell pepper, seeded and chopped
1 cup walnut halves
1 iceberg lettuce, shredded
1 handful fresh parsley, chopped

1 Mix all the ingredients, except the
   lettuce and parsley.
2 Pile the mixture on top of the lettuce.
   Sprinkle with parsley.

PEAR, AVOCADO AND NUT SALAD

SERVES 4

⅔ cup low-fat fromage blanc
Grated peel and freshly squeezed juice
   of 1 unwaxed lemon
1 tablespoon white wine vinegar
1 handful fresh chives, snipped
2 avocados, peeled, pitted, and sliced
1 pear, peeled, cored, and chopped
Salad leaves
8 walnut halves
1 handful slivered almonds

1 Mix all the ingredients, except the
   leaves and nuts; season.
2 Pile the mixture on top of the leaves
   and sprinkle with nuts.

GARLIC CHICKEN

SERVES 4

1 onion, chopped
4 celery sticks, chopped
2 carrots, chopped
1 small red bell pepper, seeded and
   chopped
1 sprig thyme
1 sprig rosemary
1 handful fresh basil leaves, torn
1 bay leaf
2 garlic bulbs, with individual cloves
   peeled but not separated from the
   bulb
4 skinless chicken breasts, about
7 ounces each
Scant ½ cup medium-dry white wine
Freshly ground black pepper
Crusty wholewheat bread, to serve
   (optional)

1 Heat the oven to 350°F.
2 Put the vegetables, herbs, and garlic
   in a baking dish. Add the chicken and
   wine and season with black pepper.
   Cover and bake 1½ hours.
3 Remove the garlic from the casserole;
   cover the casserole and keep it warm.
   Squeeze the garlic paste from the
   cloves onto slices of bread. Serve
   with the chicken.

BAKED ORIENTAL SALMON

SERVES 4

4 salmon fillets
4 scallions, shredded
1 small red bell pepper, seeded and
    thinly sliced
2-inch piece gingerroot, peeled and
    grated
1 handful fresh cilantro leaves, roughly
    chopped
4 tablespoons olive oil
Freshly squeezed juice of 1 lime
1 tablespoon low-sodium soy sauce
1 tablespoon honey (optional)
Freshly ground black pepper

1 Heat the oven to 350°F.

2 Put a large sheet of foil in a shallow
   baking dish. Lay the salmon fillets in
   a single layer in the middle. Sprinkle
   the scallions, red pepper, ginger, and
   cilantro leaves over.

3 Mix the oil, lime juice, soy sauce, and
   honey (if using). Season, then pour
   the mixture over the fish. Wrap the
   foil over the fish and seal well.

4 Bake in the oven 30 minutes, or
   until cooked. Unwrap the salmon
   and place on warm serving plates.
   Pour any juices left in the foil over
   and serve.

SALMON WITH RED PEPPER SAUTÉ

SERVES 4

4 salmon fillets
1½ teaspoons olive oil
1 small handful fresh basil, dill, or
    parsley, roughly chopped

For the red pepper sauté:
1 teaspoon olive oil
1 onion, thinly sliced
2 garlic cloves, crushed
2 red bell peppers, seeded and chopped
Scant ½ cup dry white wine
Freshly ground black pepper

1 Heat the oven to 350°F.

2 Put the salmon in a shallow baking
   dish. Brush with oil and season with
   pepper. Bake, uncovered, 20 minutes,
   or until cooked through.

3 Meanwhile, prepare the sauté. Heat
   a wok until hot. Add the oil and swirl
   it around. Stir-fry the onion and garlic
   5 minutes. Add the red pepper and
   stir-fry 5 minutes longer. Pour in the
   wine and cook for another 5 minutes,
   or until most of the liquid evaporates.

4 Divide the sauté between four plates.
   Top each with a salmon fillet.
   Sprinkle with herbs.

MEXICAN SPICED TURKEY

SERVES 4

4 tablespoons blanched almonds
6 tablespoons sesame seeds
6 tablespoons raisins
1 or 2 fresh red chilies, seeded
2 garlic cloves, crushed
2 tablepoons ground cinnamon
1 tablespoon ground cumin
1 onion, chopped
4 large tomatoes, skinned, seeded,
    and chopped
2 tablespoons olive oil
1½ cups vegetable stock (see page 153)
    or water
1 ounce dark chocolate, grated
2¼ pounds skinless turkey breast, cut
    into bite-size cubes
1 handful fresh cilantro leaves, roughly
    chopped
Freshly ground black pepper

1 Heat the oven to 350°F.

2 Toast the almonds and sesame seeds
   by tossing them in a dry skillet over
   medium heat. Grind in a blender with
   the raisins, chilies, garlic, cinnamon,
   and cumin. Add the onion and
   tomatoes and whiz in blender.

3 Heat the oil in a pan. Add the sauce
   and cook 5 minutes. Stir in the stock
   and chocolate. Season with pepper.

4 Put the turkey in a baking dish and
   pour the sauce over. Cover and bake
   45 minutes. Stir in the cilantro. Serve.

CUBAN CHICKEN

SERVES 4

4 skinless chicken breast halves
Freshly squeezed juice of 2 large
    unwaxed preferably Seville oranges,
    plus strips of peel, to serve
Freshly squeezed juice of 1 lime
1 tablespoon olive oil
2 garlic cloves, crushed
1 handful fresh herbs, such as parsley,
    cilantro, and mint, roughly chopped
1 small fresh red chili, seeded and
    finely chopped
1 handful arugula
¼ large cucumber, sliced
Freshly ground black pepper

1 Put the chicken in a single layer
   in a shallow baking dish. Mix the
   remaining ingredients, except the
   arugula and cucumber, and pour
   over the chicken; marinate 1 hour.

2 Heat the oven to 350°F.

3 Bake 25 minutes, or until cooked
   through. Serve with orange peel,
   arugula and cucumber.

HALIBUT WITH TARRAGON SAUCE

SERVES 4

1 quart vegetable stock (see page 153) or water
3¼ cups scrubbed and thickly sliced new potatoes
1 pound mixed green vegetables, such as broccoli, green beans, snow peas, sliced zucchini, and peas
⅔ cup low-fat fromage blanc
1 handful fresh tarragon, roughly chopped
Freshly ground black pepper
4 halibut fillets, about 7 ounces each

1 Heat the oven to 350°F.

2 Pour the stock into a large saucepan and bring to a boil. Add the potato and cook gently 10 minutes. Remove the potato and arrange in the base of a baking dish; reserve the stock. Scatter the green vegetables over the potatoes.

3 Mix the fromage blanc and tarragon with some of the reserved stock to make a thick sauce. Season with pepper, then pour over the vegetables. Lay the fish in a single layer on top, then cover, and bake 30 minutes. Serve.

BULGUR WHEAT WITH PEPPERS AND BEAN SPROUTS

SERVES 4

1 cup bulgur wheat
5 cups vegetable stock (page 153)
1 red bell pepper, seeded and thinly sliced
1 green bell pepper, seeded and thinly sliced
1 yellow bell pepper, seeded and thinly sliced
4 tomatoes, thinly sliced
1 handful bean sprouts
1 fresh red chili, seeded and chopped
1 handful mixed fresh herbs, such as flat-leaf parsley and mint
Grated peel and freshly squeezed juice of 1 unwaxed lemon
Freshly ground black pepper

1 Mix the ingredients in a large pan and simmer gently until the liquid is absorbed.

2 Serve hot or cold.

TROUT WITH ALMONDS AND SWEET POTATOES

SERVES 4

4 small sweet potatoes, scrubbed and
  cut into thick wedges
1 handful slivered almonds
2 tablespoons olive oil
2 tablespoons red wine vinegar
4 rainbow trout fillets, brushed with
  olive oil
Grated peel and freshly squeezed juice
  of 1 large orange
Grated peel and freshly squeezed juice
  of ½ unwaxed lemon
1 handful flat-leaf parsley, roughly
  chopped
Freshly ground black pepper

1 Heat the oven to 350°F.

2 Put the sweet potatoes, almonds, oil,
   and vinegar in a bowl and mix; season
   with black pepper. Transfer to a large
   roasting pan and bake 20 minutes.

3 Take the pan out of the oven and
   push the sweet potatoes and
   almonds to one end. Put each trout
   fillet in the middle of a piece of foil.
   Sprinkle the orange and lemon juices
   and peels over the fish, then seal in
   the foil. Put the bundles in the free
   end of the roasting pan. Return the
   pan to the oven 20 minutes, or until
   cooked.

4 Sprinkle with the chopped parsley
   and serve.

WARM MEDITERRANEAN VEGETABLE SALAD WITH BALSAMIC DRESSING

SERVES 4

For the balsamic dressing:
5 tablespoons balsamic vinegar
5 tablespoons extra virgin olive oil
1 teaspoon wholegrain mustard
3 garlic cloves, crushed
1 sprig rosemary, leaves roughly
  chopped
Freshly ground black pepper

1 red onion, cut into 8 wedges
2 zucchini, quartered lengthways
8 cherry tomatoes, cut in half
1 red bell pepper, seeded and chopped
1 yellow bell pepper, seeded and
  chopped
1 green bell pepper, seeded and chopped
9 ounces arugula or mixed baby salad
  leaves
1 handful fresh parsley, roughly chopped

1 Heat the broiler to hot.

2 Put all the dressing ingredients in a
   screw-top jar and shake.

3 Put the onion, zucchini, tomatoes,
   and peppers on a baking sheet and
   brush with a little dressing. Broil 8
   minutes until just cooked. Leave to
   cool slightly, then transfer to a large
   salad bowl.

4 Add the arugula leaves and the
   remaining dressing and toss well.
   Sprinkle the chopped parsley over
   and serve.

DESSERT RECIPES

LAMB SHANKS IN RED WINE

SERVES 4

- 2 sprigs rosemary, leaves finely chopped
- 2 garlic cloves, crushed
- 2 tablespoons olive oil
- 4 lamb shanks
- 2½ cups full-bodied red wine
- 1 onion, chopped
- 2 celery stalks, chopped
- 2 carrots, chopped
- 1 handful fresh mint leaves, roughly chopped
- Freshly ground black pepper

1 Mix the rosemary, garlic, and oil; season with pepper.

2 Put the lamb shanks in a large, deep dish. Make several deep cuts in the meat and push a little rosemary and garlic mixture into them. Spread the remaining mixture over the surface of the shanks. Pour the wine over, cover, and leave in the refrigerator to marinate at least 2 hours, preferably overnight.

3 Heat the oven to 325°F. Put the onion, celery, carrots, and mint in a baking dish. Put the lamb shanks on top and pour the marinade over. Cover and cook 1 hour. Uncover and cook 1 hour longer. Serve.

HOT BANANAS WITH PUMPKIN SEEDS & LIME

SERVES 4

- 4 bananas, chopped
- 1 handful pumpkin seeds
- 1 tablespoon shredded coconut
- 1 tablespoon honey (optional)
- Freshly squeezed juice of 1 lime
- Low-fat fromage blanc, to serve

1 Heat the oven to 350°F.

2 Mix all the ingredients, except the fromage blanc, in a baking dish. Bake 15 minutes. Serve warm with the fromage blanc.

POIRE AU CHOCOLAT
SERVES 4

4 ripe pears
8 walnut halves, chopped
1 handful slivered almonds
1 handful chopped berries, such
  as blueberries or cranberries
3½ ounces dark chocolate
4 tablespoons black decaffeinated
  coffee, cooled
4 tablespoons 2% milk (or almond, rice,
  or soymilk)

1 Peel the pears and cut a small sliver
  from the base of each so it stands
  upright. Hollow out the core from the
  base of each fruit; leave the top intact.

2 Mix together the nuts and berries
  and press some of this mixture into
  the hollow of each pear. Stand the
  stuffed pears upright in a serving dish.

3 Melt the chocolate in a heatproof
  bowl over a pan of simmering water.
  Stir in the coffee and milk. Spoon the
  mixture over the pears, then put in
  the refrigerator 2 to 3 hours. Serve
  with the remaining nut and berry
  mixture spooned over the tops.

BAKED PEACHES WITH RASPBERRIES
SERVES 4

4 large peaches
Scant ½ cup dry white wine
2 handfuls raspberries
Low-fat fromage blanc, to serve

1 Heat the oven to 350°F.

2 Put the peaches in a heatproof bowl
  and cover with boiling water; leave to
  stand 3 minutes. Remove the peaches
  and peel carefully. Cut in half and
  remove the pits. Arrange the peach
  halves, cut-side up, in a shallow
  baking dish.

3 Put 4 or 5 raspberries in the hollow
  of each peach half, with a little wine.
  Pour the rest of the wine around the
  peaches.

4 Bake 15 to 20 minutes. Serve warm
  with the fromage blanc.

BITES, SNACKS AND DRINKS

UNSWEETENED SUMMER PUDDING

SERVES 4

6 thin slices wholewheat bread, crusts removed

3 cups ripe mixed berries, such as strawberries, raspberries, blackberries, blueberries, and red currants, washed and hulled

Low-fat fromage blanc, to serve

1 Line a small pudding or mixing bowl with 4 slices of the bread—cut them into shape so they fit tightly. Put the fruit and 2 tablespoons of water in a small saucepan, gently bring to a boil over low heat, and cook 2 minutes.

2 Spoon the fruit into the bread-lined bowl, reserving the excess juice. Cover the fruit with the remaining slices of bread. Put a dish on top of the pudding and a heavy weight on top of it. Chill in the refrigerator about 8 hours.

3 Remove the weight and the dish. Put a serving plate upside-down on top of the pudding bowl and gently turn them over together, so the pudding comes out of the bowl onto the plate. Pour the reserved juice over the pudding. Serve with the fromage blanc.

GUACAMOLE

SERVES 4

1 ripe avocado, peeled and pitted

Freshly squeezed juice of ½ lemon or lime

2 teaspoons extra virgin olive oil

1 small fresh green chili

Freshly ground black pepper

1 small handful chives, snipped

Wholewheat toast, crackers, rice cakes, or crispbread

1 Put the avocado flesh, lemon or lime juice, oil, and chili in a blender. Whiz to form a smooth paste. Season with black pepper and transfer to a serving bowl. Sprinkle with the chives.

2 Spread the guacamole on the wholewheat toast, crackers, rice cakes, or crispbread, and serve.

ORANGE AND CARROT JUICE

SERVES 4

10 large oranges, peeled, pithed, and quartered

4 large carrots, peeled and chopped

1 handful crushed ice, to serve

1 Whiz the prepared oranges and carrots in a juicer. Serve with the crushed ice.

SMOKED TROUT AND LEMON PÂTÉ

SERVES 4

9 ounces smoked trout fillets
4 tablespoons low-fat yogurt with live cultures
Grated peel and freshly squeezed juice of 1 unwaxed lemon
1 handful flat-leaf parsley, roughly chopped
Freshly ground black pepper
Rye bread, rice cakes, or crispbread

1 Flake the trout and remove any bones. Mix in the yogurt, lemon juice and peel, and parsley. Season with black pepper.

2 Serve on the rye bread, rice cakes, or crispbread.

MANGO AND PAPAYA SMOOTHIE

SERVES 4

1 large mango, flesh roughly chopped
1 papaya, flesh roughly chopped
2½ cups 2% milk (or almond, rice, or soymilk)
⅔ cup low-fat yogurt with live cultures
1 handful crushed ice

1 Put all the ingredients in a blender and whiz until smooth. Serve immediately.

VEGETABLE STOCK

MAKES ABOUT 3 QUARTS

6 carrots, roughly chopped
3 onions, roughly chopped
3 leeks, roughly chopped
3 celery sticks, roughly chopped
1 bunch green leaves, such as lettuce
6 sprigs parsley, including stems
3 sprigs thyme
1 sprig rosemary
1 bay leaf
6 black peppercorns
3½ quarts water

1 Put all the ingredients in a large pan, cover, and bring to a boil; skim off any scum. Simmer gently 1 hour.

2 Cool slightly, then strain. Don't force solids through the strainer unless you want cloudy stock.

INTRODUCING THE MODERATE PROGRAM

The moderate program is more advanced than the gentle program. It's ideal for people who have completed the gentle program and wish to move on, or for those who want greater blood pressure-lowering benefits than those provided by the gentle program. You need to be relatively fit and healthy, and you probably already eat healthily with plenty of fresh fruit and vegetables.

There are 14 daily plans that you can repeat to create a 28-day program. Follow the program for at least a month before assessing its benefits. Once you feel comfortable with the diet and lifestyle changes involved, feel free to make your own adjustments that take into account your tastes and lifestyle.

THE MODERATE PROGRAM DIET

The daily food plans in this program are based on a low–glycemic index (GI) diet. As well as following the principles of the Dietary Approaches to Stop Hypertension (DASH; see page 66), the diet includes more of the superfoods that are particularly beneficial for people with hypertension (see pages 80–86). There are a greater number of vegetarian and fish dishes than in the gentle program, and I also introduce you to home-sprouted beans and seeds, homemade fruit and vegetable juices, and a wider variety of grains than you might have eaten previously.

This diet has the potential to lower blood pressure by 7/4–11/5 mmHg or more within 30 days, even if you're taking anti-hypertensive medications. This style of eating will also lower your total and LDL-cholesterol levels and reduce your triglyceride levels (see page 50).

As part of the moderate program you can eat a daily 1½-ounce piece of dark chocolate (at least 70 percent cocoa solids) and drink up to ⅔ cup red wine per day if you wish. Unsweetened red grape juice provides an alternative source of antioxidants for those who prefer not to drink alcohol on a regular basis.

SPROUTING BEANS AND SEEDS

I recommend you start sprouting your own beans and seeds during the program. You can do this easily in a jam jar, but you can also buy a customized germinator, which provides the correct conditions of warmth and humidity for optimal growth. Homesprouted beans and seeds are a great source of vitamins, minerals, trace elements, and live enzymes. You can add them to salads, stir-fries, rice, soups, and all kinds of chicken, fish, and vegetarian dishes.

Simply rinse 4 to 6 tablespoons mixed organic beans or seeds in water. Put in a glass jar or sprinkle lightly over a germinator, and leave to germinate for three to five days. Choose any of the following: alfalfa, radish, broccoli, white radish, red clover, mustard and cress seeds, wheat, lentils, quinoa, or mung beans.

SHOPPING LIST

You will need all the food and drink items on the shopping list for the gentle program (see page 114). In addition you will need the following (whenever possible, buy regularly in small quantities for optimum freshness).

DRINKS
decaffeinated coffee, rosé wine, vanilla rooibos tea

DAIRY AND SOY PRODUCTS
firm tofu, silken tofu

FRUIT AND VEGETABLES
bean sprouts and seeds for sprouting, beets, black olives (unsalted), butternut squash, fennel, grape leaves, pomegranate, prunes, radicchio, wild mushrooms

NUTS AND SEEDS
(Always choose unsalted varieties), cashew nuts, hazelnuts, pine nuts, poppy seeds

HERBS AND SAUCES
lemongrass, low-sodium pesto sauce

GRAINS
couscous, hemp pasta, quinoa, red rice, spinach or wholewheat lasagne sheets, wild rice, steel-cut oats

PROTEINS
black beans, crab, shrimp, sea bass,

MISCELLANEOUS
rosewater

MAKING YOUR OWN JUICES

I also suggest you invest in a juicer so you can start making your own juices. Freshly prepared juice has a creamy texture, a milky hue, and is richer in vitamins and antioxidants than juice that has sat on a shelf or in a refrigerator several days. Although you will remove much of the insoluble fiber from the fruit or vegetables when juicing, you obtain significantly more vitamins and minerals than when eating fruit and vegetables in their natural raw state. The secret is in their concentration. One 3½-ounce glass carrot juice can give you as much betacarotene as about 1 pound raw carrots. Here are some tips for making delicious juices at home:

- Pick garden-fresh fruit and vegetables. As soon as they are harvested, vitamin content drops.
- If possible, buy organic produce that has not come into contact with artificial fertilizers or pesticides.
- Choose firm, plump produce with a good color.
- Citrus fruit with tough skins need peeling before juicing, but you can process lemons and limes intact for flavor.
- Choose seedless varieties of grape and remove the stems to avoid a bitter taste.
- Some fruits, such as bananas and avocado, can be difficult to juice —they are best mashed or blended and then stirred into other fruit juice bases.
- Virtually any blend of fruit, vegetable, or herb is possible—experiment.
- Dilute juice with mineral water for a thirst-quenching drink. Milk can also be added to some juices, such as carrot juice.

EATING A VARIETY OF GRAINS

Some of the grains in the moderate program might be unfamiliar to you, so here's a brief guide to hemp pasta, red rice, wild rice, and quinoa. Hemp pasta, made from flour and oil derived from hemp seeds (related to sunflower seeds), have a similar protein content to soybeans, but are also a rich source of omega-3 oils and vitamin E.

Red rice (such as from the Camargue or Bhutan) has a nutty flavor and a chewy texture. It has the same nutritional value as brown rice, but cooks twice as quickly. Wild rice is the seed of a water grass. It's fermented to make it easier to hull and to improve its nutty flavor. It's often mixed with brown or red rice.

Quinoa is the seed of a plant related to spinach. It's an excellent source of protein (50 percent higher than most grains), vitamin E, and B-group vitamins and folate, as well as minerals such as potassium, magnesium, zinc, copper, and manganese.

FOODS TO AVOID OR EAT LESS OF

As I recommend in the gentle program, throw away any foods in your cupboards that are high in sugar, salt, saturated fat, and trans fats. Do not be tempted to add salt during cooking or at the table. Obtain flavor from fresh herbs and black pepper instead.

THE MODERATE PROGRAM EXERCISE ROUTINE

The moderate exercise program is designed for those who are relatively fit and who already exercise regularly for 30 minutes on most days of the week. Over the course of the program you will increase the amount of time you exercise. You will also do weight exercises to complement the aerobic exercise you're taking. In the second half of the program I introduce qigong (see pages 62–63). As well as improving physical well-being, qigong has the power to calm your mind.

When starting an exercise program, always monitor your 10-second pulse rate (see pages 101–102). If you have angina or a history of heart attack, ask your doctor for guidance on how much exercise you can take.

THE MODERATE PROGRAM THERAPIES

In this program I introduce you to several complementary therapies that can help to reduce your blood pressure. You will find straightforward relaxation techniques to practice on many days of the program. Please look at days seven, thirteen, and fourteen of the program so you can book appointments with the therapists I advise you to see.

MODERATE PROGRAM SUPPLEMENTS

The supplements I suggest you take when following the moderate program are similar to those in the gentle program, but, when appropriate, at a higher, more therapeutic dose. You can find information about these supplements and their blood-pressure-lowering effects on pages 86–92.

Recommended daily supplements

- Vitamin C (1,000 mg)
- Vitamin E (400 i.u/268 mg)
- Lycopene carotenoid complex (15 mg)
- Selenium (100 mcg)
- Coenzyme Q10 (90 mg)
- Garlic tablets (allicin yield 1,000 mcg–1,500 mcg)
- Omega-3 fish oil (600 mg daily; for example, 2x1g fish oil capsules, each supplying 180 mg eicosapentaenoic acid, EPA, plus 120 mg docosahexaenoic acid, DHA)

Optional daily supplements (these will provide additional health benefits)

- Alpha-lipoic acid (200 mg). May be combined with L-carnitine in a 1:1 ratio
- Magnesium (300 mg)
- Calcium (800 mg)
- Folic acid (600 mcg) plus vitamin B12 (50mcg)
- Reishi (1,000 mg)
- Bilberry fruit extracts (120 mg—standardized to give 25 percent anthocyanins)
- Probiotics (fermented milk drinks, yogurt with live cultures, or supplements)

THE MODERATE PROGRAM
DAY ONE

DAILY MENU

Breakfast: homemade muesli (see page 141) with chopped almonds and berries
Morning snack: a piece of fruit (choose from the selection on the shopping list; see page 114)
Lunch: ½ avocado. Bowl of mixed salad leaves sprinkled with 1 tablespoon seeds and balsamic dressing (see page 149). Low-fat yogurt with live cultures with blueberries
Afternoon snack: a handful of almonds
Dinner: mushroom and walnut lasagne (see page 193). Broccoli. Baby carrots. About 1½ ounces dark chocolate
Drinks: 2½ cups 2% or 1% milk. Freshly squeezed fruit/veg juice. Unlimited green, black, white, or herbal tea, and mineral water. 5 ounces (⅔ cup) red wine or unsweetened red grape juice
Supplements: see page 158

DAILY EXERCISE ROUTINE

During the first week of this program, I will set muscle-toning exercises that build up into a daily strength and suppleness regime. This is important to prepare you for your slowly increasing level of physical activity. Start with seated leg lifts, which work the muscles in the fronts of your thighs. In addition to the muscle-toning exercises, walk for 30 minutes at a moderate to brisk pace.

SEATED LEG LIFTS

1 Sit up straight on the edge of your bed, with your feet flat on the floor and your hands on the bed by your sides.
2 Extend your left leg until it's straight out in front of you.
3 Hold for a count of three, then slowly lower it.
4 Do this 10 times. Repeat with your right leg.

YOGA BREATHING

Over the next few days I will explain some key yogic breathing techniques, known as pranayama. Today's technique is known as dirgha—the three-part breath. It is perhaps the most important yogic pranayama because it overcomes the modern affliction of shallow breathing.

DIRGHA—THE THREE-PART BREATH

1 Sit comfortably in a cross-legged position, with your back straight. Close your eyes and, as you breathe in and out, focus on the expansion and contraction of your ribcage.

2 Breathe into the lower part of your ribcage and, with each exhalation, allow all tension to flow away.

3 Now breathe into your lower ribcage and then draw more breath in so the middle part of your ribcage expands.

4 Continue inhaling. Make the third part of your in-breath expand the upper part of your lungs—feel your clavicles (collar bones) rise up.

5 Breathe smoothly in this way for 5 minutes or as long you want to. If you feel light-headed, stop. End by breathing normally for 10 minutes in quiet contemplation. Carry the sense of calm you have gained into your day.

DAY TWO

DAILY MENU

Breakfast: oatmeal with sliced apple
Morning snack: a piece of fruit
Lunch: bowl of sliced green, yellow, and red bell peppers, sprouted beans, celery, and mixed salad leaves sprinkled with balsamic dressing (see page 149). Wholewheat or hemp pasta. Low-fat yogurt with live cultures with black or red grapes
Afternoon snack: a handful of walnuts
Dinner: salmon steak baked with lemon, garlic, and dill. Steamed green beans drizzled with almond oil. Brown, red, or wild rice, or quinoa. Baked banana with low-fat fromage blanc
Drinks: 2½ cups 2% or 1% milk. Freshly squeezed fruit/veg juice. Unlimited green, black, white, or herbal tea, and mineral water. 5 ounces (⅔ cup) red wine or unsweetened red grape juice
Supplements: see page 158

Today's dinnertime dessert is baked banana—in Ayurvedic medicine bananas are used to help lower blood pressure. They are a good source of potassium and also have an angiotensin–converting enzyme (ACE) blocking action (highest in ripe bananas).

DAILY EXERCISE ROUTINE

Walk at a moderate to brisk pace for 30 minutes today. Do your muscle-toning exercise from day one, followed by these seated squats, which tone your arms and legs. To do the squats you will need two small weights of about 1 pound each. These can be either cans of food or dumbbells.

SEATED SQUATS

1 Sit on the edge of your bed, so your toes are below your knees and your feet and knees are shoulder-width apart.
2 Hold a weight in each hand, and place your elbows by your sides so the backs of your hands rest lightly on the bed.
3 Take a deep breath in and, as you breathe out, slowly stand up, curling the weights up to your shoulders.
4 Take a deep breath in and, as you breathe out, slowly sit back down while lowering your arms. Do this as slowly as possible, feeling the contraction in your muscles. Repeat 10 times.

YOGA BREATHING

Today's pranayama can be carried out on almost any occasion, without anyone noticing.

LENGTHENING YOUR OUT-BREATH

1 Sit comfortably, with your arms hanging loosely by your sides. Slowly inhale until your lungs are full of air. Focus on the rise of your abdomen rather than your chest. Breathe out and try to empty your lungs of air.
2 Gradually speed up your inhalations, and slow down your exhalations until you spend 3 seconds breathing in, and 7 seconds breathing out.
3 Keep breathing like this at a rate of just six breaths per minute (half the normal rate). Focus on emptying your lungs, and on keeping air flow continuous—don't hold your breath between inhaling and exhaling. Do this for 5 minutes.

DAY THREE

DAILY MENU

Breakfast: low-fat fromage blanc mixed with chopped almonds and blueberries
Morning snack: piece of fruit
Lunch: cream of watercress soup (see page 185). Bowl of mixed salad leaves sprinkled with mixed nuts, sprouted beans, dill, grated beet, and balsamic dressing (see page 149). Crackers. Low-fat yogurt with live cultures with black grapes
Afternoon snack: a handful of almonds
Dinner: roasted red peppers with herby bulgur wheat (see page 191). Bowl of mixed salad leaves sprinkled with mixed nuts. Tropical fruit salad
Drinks: 2½ cups 2% or 1% milk. Freshly squeezed fruit/veg juice. Unlimited green, black, white, or herbal tea, and mineral water. 5 ounces (⅔ cup) red wine or unsweetened red grape juice
Supplements: see page 158

As you do your brisk walk today, remind yourself that this one session of moderately intense exercise can lower your blood pressure for up to 24 hours. After three consecutive days of exercise, your blood pressure is reduced for longer. Three out of four people with hypertension show benefits when starting a regular exercise program, with an average blood pressure reduction of 11/8 mmHg. Blood pressure returns to pre-exercise levels after one to two weeks of no exercise.

DAILY EXERCISE ROUTINE

Walk at a moderate to brisk pace for 30 minutes today. Do your muscle-toning exercises from days one and two, followed by the seated bridge, which tones your back, leg, and arm muscles.

SEATED BRIDGE

1 Sit on the edge of your bed, with your feet flat on the floor and your knees bent at 90 degrees. Rest your palms on the edge of the bed by your sides, fingers facing forward.
2 Take a deep breath in and, as you breathe out, lift your hips so your weight is supported by your palms and feet. Continue lifting your body

and arch your back up until you're in a bridge shape. Hold for 20 seconds (while breathing normally), then slowly sit back down.

YOGA BREATHING

Today's breathing exercise improves your focus and promotes a sense of power and oneness.

UJJAYI—OCEAN BREATH

1 Sit comfortably in a cross-legged position on the floor. Breathe deeply in and out through your mouth. Start to make a soft, whispering, haaaaahhhh noise as you breathe out, by slightly constricting the back of your throat—as if you were trying to fog up a window.

2 Do this several times on your out-breath. When you're comfortable doing this, make the same noise as you inhale. Your breathing should sound like the ebb and flow of the ocean.

3 Now practice the same breath again but through your nose. Do this for a few minutes.

DAY FOUR

DAILY MENU

Breakfast: homemade muesli (see page 141) with dates

Morning snack: a piece of fruit

Lunch: smoked mackerel and mango medley (see page 186). Wholewheat roll. Low-fat yogurt with live cultures with fresh fruit

Afternoon snack: a handful of walnuts

Dinner: stir-fried turkey with bean sprouts (see page 192). Bok choy. Red, brown, or wild rice, or quinoa. About 1½ ounces dark chocolate

Drinks: 2½ cups 2% or 1% milk. Freshly squeezed

fruit/veg juice. Unlimited green, black, white, or herbal tea, and mineral water. 5 ounces (⅔ cup) red wine or unsweetened red grape juice

Supplements: see page 158

DAILY EXERCISE ROUTINE

Walk at a moderate to brisk pace for 30 minutes today. Do your muscle-toning exercises from days one through three, followed by this seated triceps dip to tone your upper arms.

SEATED TRICEPS DIP

1 Sit on the very edge of a bed, with your knees bent and your feet flat on the floor. Place your hands on the edge of the bed, fingers facing forward.
2 Keep your arms straight and lift your bottom off the edge of the bed. Keeping your back straight and your stomach muscles pulled in, bend your elbows and lower your bottom toward the ground. Make sure your elbows don't pivot outward by slightly squeezing them in toward each other.
3 Straighten your arms to lift your hips again. Repeat five times.

YOGA BREATHING

Today's breathing exercise teaches you how to interrupt your inhalations. It serves as an introduction to tomorrow's exercise, which lowers blood pressure. You need only practice today's exercise on this occasion—I have included it so you can familarize yourself with the technique.

VILOMA PRANAYAMA STAGE 1

1 Spend 5 minutes relaxing quietly in corpse pose (see page 136) with your eyes closed.
2 Breathe in for 2 to 3 seconds, then hold your breath for 2 to 3 seconds. Breathe in for another 2 to 3 seconds, then hold your breath again. Repeat until your lungs are full (normally four to five mini-breaths).
3 Now breathe out slowly and steadily until your lungs feel empty. Breathe normally before repeating the exercise once more. Spend some time resting in quiet contemplation before getting up.

CALMING BREATH
Research shows that yogic breathing promotes reduced oxygen consumption, decreased heart rate, and lowered blood pressure.

DAY FIVE

DAILY MENU

Breakfast: spicy garlic mushrooms (see page 183)
Morning snack: a piece of fruit
Lunch: soused herring (see page 187). Bowl of mixed salad leaves sprinkled with mixed seeds and walnut oil. Wholewheat roll.

Low-fat yogurt with live cultures. Kiwi
Afternoon snack: a handful of almonds
Dinner: cinnamon eggplant (see page 189). Spinach. Corn kernels. Wholewheat or hemp pasta. Oat flummery (see page 194)

Drinks: 2½ cups 2% or 1% milk. Freshly squeezed fruit/veg juice. Unlimited green, black, white, or herbal tea, and mineral water. 5 ounces (⅔ cup) red wine or unsweetened red grape juice
Supplements: see page 158

Today's main meal contains eggplant, a vegetable believed to help reduce cholesterol levels partly through antioxidant action, and partly by stimulating bile production in the liver so more cholesterol is excreted. Although recipes often suggest using salt to draw out the bitter juices from eggplant, I don't advise this. Salting is highly unsuitable for anyone with hypertension; and the bitter ingredients give eggplant its important health benefits.

DAILY EXERCISE ROUTINE

Walk at a moderate to brisk pace for 30 minutes today. Do your muscle-toning exercises from days one through four, followed by kneeling leg lifts, which tone your buttocks and the backs of your thighs.

KNEELING LEG LIFTS

1 Kneel on all fours with your head slightly down, and your back straight and parallel to the floor.
2 Extend one leg back so it's completely straight behind you. Hold for a count of three, then return to kneeling on all fours.
3 Do 10 of these with each leg.

YOGA BREATHING

Viloma pranayama stage 2 is an advanced breathing exercise used to reduce hypertension. Its rhythm is easier to understand once you have tried yesterday's interrupted breathing exercise.

VILOMA PRANAYAMA STAGE 2

1 Spend 5 minutes resting quietly in corpse pose (see page 136) with your eyes closed.
2 When you feel ready, exhale completely until your lungs feel empty. Then inhale smoothly until your lungs feel full.
3 Exhale slowly for 2 or 3 seconds, then pause, holding your breath for 2 to 3 seconds. Exhale further for 2 to 3 seconds before pausing again. Repeat until your lungs feel empty (usually four to five pauses).
4 Breathe in and out normally a few times, then repeat.
5 Do between five and 10 interrupted exhalations. With practice, you can spend 10 minutes alternating interrupted exhalations with three cycles of normal breathing. To finish, lie quietly, and breathe normally.

DAY SIX

DAILY MENU

Breakfast: homemade muesli (see page 141) with added almonds, flax seeds, and berries
Morning snack: a piece of fruit
Lunch: chickpea and avocado hummus (see page 195). Bowl of mixed salad leaves sprinkled with mixed seeds, sprouted beans, and balsamic dressing (see page 149). Low-fat yogurt with live cultures with fresh fruit
Afternoon snack: a handful of walnuts
Dinner: roast tomato and red pepper soup (see page 187). Broiled, skinless chicken breasts marinated in olive oil and lime juice. Broccoli. Red, brown, or wild rice, or quinoa
Drinks: 2½ cups 2% or 1% milk. Freshly squeezed fruit/veg juice. Unlimited green, black, white, or herbal tea, and mineral water. 5 ounces (²⁄₃ cup) red wine or unsweetened red grape juice
Supplements: see page 158

Removing the skin from chicken and other poultry makes your meal healthier. Tonight's meal would contain ½ ounce fat per 3½-ounce serving with the skin on the chicken breast, but only ⁷⁄₁₀₀ ounce per 3½-ounce serving without the skin.

DAILY EXERCISE ROUTINE

Having walked every day this week, I suggest you now start a cycling regime. Ideally, cycle every other day, and walk on those days when you're not cycling. You can cycle outdoors (make sure you wear a helmet) or on a fixed exercise bike. Do your muscle-toning exercises from days one through five, followed by kneeling leg raises, which work on your upper thighs and buttocks.

KNEELING LEG RAISES

1 Kneel on all fours with your head slightly down, and your back parallel to the floor.
2 Extend your right leg straight out behind you. Bend your right knee to 90 degrees, so the sole of your foot is parallel to the ceiling. Using small movements, lift your right foot up and down 10 times.
3 Lower your leg back down to the starting position. Repeat the exercise three times. Repeat with your left leg.

YOGA BREATHING

Today's technique promotes quietness and is used therapeutically for people with hypertension.

ALTERNATE NOSTRIL BREATHING

1 Sit comfortably with your back straight (cross-legged on the floor is ideal).
2 When you feel ready, close your right nostril with your thumb. Breathe in through your left nostril, slowly and deeply while counting to four.
3 Release your right nostril and use your ring and little fingers to close your left nostril. Now breathe out through your right nostril while counting to eight.

4 Breathe in through the right nostril to a count of four.

5 Release the left nostril, close the right nostril with your thumb and exhale through the left nostril to a count of eight. Do this cycle twice at first. Work up to 10 repetitions. End with quiet contemplation.

DAY SEVEN

DAILY MENU

Breakfast: vanilla rooibos compote (see page 183). Low-fat yogurt with live cultures

Morning snack: a piece of fruit

Lunch: cream of watercress soup (see page 185). Bowl of mixed salad leaves sprinkled with mixed seeds, bean sprouts, grated beet, chopped mint, and balsamic dressing (see page 149). Whole-wheat roll or pita bread. Low-fat yogurt with fresh fruit

Afternoon snack: a handful of almonds

Dinner: mushroom and walnut lasagne (see page 193). Spinach. Baby carrots. Creamy Turkish delight figs (see page 195)

Drinks: 2½ cups 2% or 1% milk. Freshly squeezed fruit/veg juice. Unlimited green, black, white, or herbal tea, and mineral water. 5 ounces (⅔ cup) red wine or unsweetened red grape juice

Supplements: see page 158

DAILY EXERCISE ROUTINE

Go for a brisk 35-minute walk today. Do your muscle-toning exercises from days one through six, followed by plank raises, which tone your arms and abdominals.

PLANK RAISES

1 Lie face down on the floor with your arms bent and hands flat on the floor near your shoulders ready to do a press-up. Press your toes into the ground, pull in your abdominal muscle and straighten your arms to lift your body into a straight, planklike line from your heels to your head.

2 Stay in the plank position for 3 seconds, then slowly lower yourself to the ground. Do this five times.

CONSULTING A MEDICAL HERBALIST

Now that this first week is over, I suggest that you visit a medical herbalist who will select the herbal remedies most likely to suit you as an individual. In the first consultation, which usually lasts one hour, an herbalist will assess your general health and ask about any medicines and supplements you're taking. He or she will ask you about your diet, work, lifestyle, medical history, and current physical, mental, and emotional state. An herbalist will examine your pulse and might listen to your heart and lungs. He or she will give you one or more herbal remedies to take away. Herbs are often prescribed as tinctures (made by steeping herbs in alcohol) or as decoctions (in which herbs are boiled in water). Herbal tablets and capsules are also used. The results of treatment are assessed in 15 to 30-minute followups. As a guide, expect to need a month of treatment for every year you have had hypertension. To find an herbalist, see page 237.

DAY EIGHT

DAILY MENU

Breakfast: banana-cinnamon oatmeal (see page 141)
Morning snack: a piece of fruit
Lunch: bowl of chopped avocado and tomatoes mixed with sprouted beans, pomegranate, and radicchio in a balsamic dressing (see page 149).

Wholewheat roll. Low-fat yogurt with live cultures with fresh fruit
Afternoon snack: a handful of walnuts
Dinner: mock caviar (see page 196). Salmon steak marinated in olive oil and lime juice and baked. Red, brown, or wild rice, or quinoa.

Spinach with olive oil
Drinks: 2½ cups 2% or 1% milk. Freshly squeezed fruit/veg juice. Unlimited green, black, white, or herbal tea, and mineral water. 5 ounces (⅔ cup) red wine or unsweetened red grape juice
Supplements: see page 158

DAILY EXERCISE ROUTINE

Go for a brisk 35-minute walk today, or cycle for 20 minutes. Do your muscle-toning exercises from days one through seven. Today, I introduce a sequence of qigong exercises (see pages 62–63) that will help you wind down at the end of the day. The opening position will prepare your mind and body for the sequence. Return to this posture between each qigong exercise.

QIGONG OPENING POSITION

1 Stand straight with your feet close together and touching, toes pointing forward. Let your arms relax at your sides with your palms facing inward. Unlock your knees.
2 Relax your body—imagine you are a puppet on a string. Keep your head up, looking forward. Part your lips and lightly touch the roof of your mouth with the tip of your tongue. Breathe gently in through your nose and out through your mouth.

MEDITATION

From today onward, spend 15 minutes a day in quiet meditation/ visualization—this is a powerful tool that can significantly reduce your blood pressure. Here is the first meditation.

THE INNER SMILE

1 Sit or stand comfortably and practice one of the breathing techniques you have learned. Now imagine something that makes you smile. Allow the smile to shine out of your eyes and travel inward.
2 Focus on your navel area. Let the smile radiate here. Become relaxed and calm. See if you can feel a warmth or vibration in the pit of your stomach.

MUSIC THERAPY
Research shows that classical music can relax you, which is good for your blood pressure. In one study, one group of people listened to Mozart, another group listened to new age music, and a third group read magazines. After three days, those listening to Mozart reported the highest levels of peacefulness, mental quiet, and relaxation.

DAY NINE

DAILY MENU

Breakfast: figs with pomegranate (see page 184)
Morning snack: a piece of fruit
Lunch: black bean compote with cumin and cilantro (see page 185). Bowl of mixed salad leaves sprinkled with mixed seeds and drizzled with walnut oil. Wholewheat roll.

Low-fat yogurt with live cultures with fruit
Afternoon snack: toasted mixed nuts (see page 195)
Dinner: stuffed grape leaves with tzatziki (see page 190). Bowl of mixed salad leaves sprinkled with black olives and mixed seeds in a balsamic dressing (see page 149).

Mulled fruit salad (see page 194)
Drinks: 2½ cups 2% or 1% milk. Freshly squeezed fruit/veg juice. Unlimited green, black, white, or herbal tea, and mineral water. 5 ounces (⅔ cup) red wine or unsweetened red grape juice
Supplements: see page 158

DAILY EXERCISE ROUTINE

Go for a brisk 35-minute walk today, or cycle for 20 minutes. Do your muscle-toning exercises from days one through seven. In the evening practice the qigong posture from day eight, and then do the following exercise, which opens the heart and lungs and encourages the free flow of qi.

QIGONG—OPENING THE HEART

1 In the opening position, breathe in and raise your arms in front of you to shoulder height. As you breathe out, make a breast-stroke movement: extend your arms to the sides, bend your elbows, and bring your hands together in front of your chest.

2 Continue this movement for 1 minute. Then stand in contemplation for 1 minute.

VISUALIZATION

This powerful visualization will help to lower your blood pressure.

BLUE LIGHT VISUALIZATION

1 Sit quietly with your eyes closed. Imagine your body as a pulsating, red shape.

STRESS-BUSTING

Stress makes hypertension worse, so it's important to pinpoint the causes of stress and tackle them. Common causes are relationship or work problems or feeling that there is "never enough time." Try to learn time management skills, and how to prioritize tasks and delegate. Pace yourself—make time for exercise and meals. Take regular breaks. Try to separate work from home and learn how to be assertive so you're effective at expressing your needs. If self-help techniques don't work, consider going on a stress-management course or seeing a stress counselor.

2 Imagine a light bulb is switched on above you. It gives out healing blue light that bathes your body and enters your cells.

3 Visualize your pulsating red shape change to a gentle, undulating blue form. Bask in the cool, restful glow as the blue light lowers your blood pressure. Relax in the light for 15 minutes.

DAY TEN

DAILY MENU

Breakfast: homemade muesli (see page 141)
Morning snack: a piece of fruit
Lunch: warm chickpea salad (see page 186). Bowl of mixed salad leaves sprinkled with mixed nuts, grated beet, and extra virgin olive oil.

Low-fat yogurt with live cultures with fresh fruit
Afternoon snack: a handful of walnuts
Dinner: rosé trout (see page 193). Broccoli. Sweet potatoes. Corn kernels. Oat flummery (see page 194)

Drinks: 2½ cups 2% or 1% milk. Freshly squeezed fruit/veg juice. Unlimited green, black, white, or herbal tea, and mineral water. 5 ounces (²⁄₃ cup) red wine or unsweetened red grape juice
Supplements: see page 158

Today's dinner is trout cooked in rosé wine; trout contains a useful amount of omega-3 fatty acids, while the addition of almonds and wine increases the antioxidant value and cholesterol-lowering properties of this tasty dish.

DAILY EXERCISE ROUTINE

Go for a brisk 35-minute walk today or cycle for 20 minutes. Do your muscle-toning exercises from days one through seven. In the evening, practice the qigong exercises from days eight and nine, and then do the following exercise.

QIGONG—DIRECTING QI INTERNALLY

1 Stand in the opening position. Rub your hands together, then place your hands on the base of your ribcage—your right hand on the right side and your left hand on the left. Move your hands in a circle and visualize qi flowing from your hands into your liver on the right and your spleen on the left.
2 Feel the heat welling up in your hands and traveling into your body, helping your internal organs to function.
3 Move your hands over your sternum and navel. Visualize qi passing from your hands into your heart and major blood vessels. Finally, move your palms to your lower back and visualize qi flowing into your kidneys and adrenal glands.
4 Continue for as long as you feel qi flowing strongly, then return to the opening position.

ACUPRESSURE

This acupressure technique will help you relax. Find your third eye point—between your eyebrows on the bridge of your nose. Massage this point firmly with your dominant middle finger. Make small rotating movements, both clockwise and anticlockwise, to reduce an excess of stagnant qi. Manipulate this point for 3 minutes to help clear and calm your mind.

BIKE POWER
As you get fitter, you can slowly increase the intensity of your cycling by pedaling faster or riding up hills.

DAY ELEVEN

DAILY MENU

Breakfast: raspberry and Brazil nut medley (see page 184)
Morning snack: a piece of fruit
Lunch: cream of watercress soup (see page 185). Wholewheat roll. Low-fat yogurt with fruit.
Afternoon snack: berry smoothie (see page 196)
Dinner: broiled mushrooms with almonds and basil (see page 194). Roasted vegetables (baby vine tomatoes, zucchini, eggplant, red bell pepper, and red onion). Wholewheat or hemp pasta. About 1½ ounces dark chocolate
Drinks: 2½ cups 2% or 1% milk. Freshly squeezed fruit/veg juice. Unlimited green, black, white, or herbal tea, and mineral water. 5 ounces (⅔ cup) red wine or unsweetened red grape juice
Supplements: see page 158

DAILY EXERCISE ROUTINE

Go for a brisk 40-minute walk today, or cycle for 25 minutes. Do your muscle-toning exercises from days one through seven. In the evening, practice the qigong exercises from days eight through ten, and then do the following exercise, which directs qi down through your body to promote a sense of calm and improve your circulation.

QIGONG—DIRECTING QI DOWNWARD

1 Stand in the opening position. Breathe in deeply. Raise your arms and bring your palms together in a prayerlike gesture in front of your upper chest.

2 Carefully raise your left leg and bend it so your left ankle rests on your right knee. As you breathe out, gently bend your right leg and let your weight sink into it. Maintain your balance here for 30 to 60 seconds; repeat with the other leg. Return to the opening position for quiet contemplation.

MUSCLE RELAXATION

Close the curtains, light some candles, and play some classical music for this relaxation exercise.

TENSION SCAN

At various points in your day, stop and mentally scan your body for areas of muscle tension. Are you carrying tension in your back, shoulder, or jaw muscles? If so, make a point of releasing that tension.

PROGRESSIVE MUSCLE RELAXATION 1

1 Lie down on a mat or bed, close your eyes, and breathe slowly and deeply. Begin by clenching your toes. Hold for a count of 10, then relax. Feel the tension drop away.

2 Flex your feet. Hold for a count of 10 then release and let the tension go.

3 Move slowly up your body, through your legs, buttocks, abdomen, back, shoulders, arms, hands, fingers, neck, and head, clenching then relaxing each group of muscles.

4 Keep checking back on the muscles you have worked on to make sure tension has not crept back into them. Once your whole body is relaxed, lie quietly for 10 minutes.

DAY TWELVE

DAILY MENU

Breakfast: spicy garlic mushrooms (see page 183)
Morning snack: a piece of fruit
Lunch: bowl of mixed salad leaves sprinkled with mixed seeds, grated beet, and walnut oil. Wholewheat pita bread or mixed-grain roll. Low-fat

yogurt with live cultures with fresh fruit
Afternoon snack: a handful of walnuts
Dinner: French onion soup (see page 188). Skinless chicken or turkey piece, marinated in olive oil and fresh herbs, then broiled. Spinach. Couscous

Drinks: 2½ cups 2% or 1% milk. Freshly squeezed fruit/veg juice. Unlimited green, black, white, or herbal tea, and mineral water. 5 ounces (⅔ cup) red wine or unsweetened red grape juice
Supplements: see page 158

Today's French onion soup is a delicious and nutritious start to your dinner. Onions contain similar sulfur-containing phytochemicals to garlic (see page 83).

DAILY EXERCISE ROUTINE

Go for a brisk 40-minute walk today, or cycle for 25 minutes. Do your muscle-toning exercises from days one through seven. In the evening, wind down with the qigong sequence from days eight through eleven, then do the following.

QIGONG—BALANCING BLOOD PRESSURE

1 Stand in the opening position. Stretch your right arm out to the side so it's parallel to the floor, palm facing upward. Now arch your left arm up to form a gentle curve, with your palm facing the top of your head.
2 Move your weight onto your left leg, bending your knee slightly. Keep your right leg straight and raise your right heel slightly. Turn your head to look at your right hand.
3 Now arch your right arm overhead and stretch your left arm out to the side, palm facing up. At the same time, move your weight onto your right leg, bending slightly at the knee. Straighten your left leg and let your left heel rise slightly. Turn to look to the left.
4 Move gently from side to side in this way, several times.

RELAXATION

Today's technique is similar to yesterday's, but promotes a deeper level of muscle awareness.

PROGRESSIVE MUSCLE RELAXATION 2

1 Lie down, close your eyes, and breathe deeply. Bend your toes slightly so just a little tension enters them. Count to 10, then relax—feel tension drop away.
2 Flex your feet slightly. Hold for a count of 10 then release—feel the tension go.
3 Work your way up your body minimally tightening each group of muscles then relaxing them. Be aware of how a slightly tensed muscle feels different from a fully relaxed muscle.
4 Finish by minimally tensing every muscle in your body at the same time, then let go.

DAY THIRTEEN

DAILY MENU

Breakfast: figs with pomegranate (see page 184)
Morning snack: a piece of fruit
Lunch: smoked mackerel and mango medley (see page 186). Bowl of mixed salad leaves sprinkled with sprouting beans, grated beet, and fennel, mixed seeds and walnut oil. Low-fat yogurt with live cultures
Afternoon snack: a handful of almonds
Dinner: stir-fried bean sprouts, carrots, scallions, mushrooms, sugarsnap peas, and broccoli, with ginger, garlic, cilantro, and lemongrass. Red, brown, or wild rice, or quinoa. Stewed, unsweetened rhubarb with low-fat vanilla fromage blanc
Drinks: 2½ cups 2% or 1% milk. Freshly squeezed fruit/veg juice. Unlimited green, black, white, or herbal tea, and mineral water. 5 ounces (⅔ cup) red wine or unsweetened red grape juice
Supplements: see page 158

DAILY EXERCISE ROUTINE

Go for a brisk 40-minute walk or cycle for 25 minutes today. Do your muscle-toning exercises from days one through seven. In the evening, wind down with the qigong sequence from days eight through twelve, then add the following exercise, which removes stagnant qi and replenishes it with fresh, universal qi.

QIGONG—REMOVING STAGNANT QI

1 Stand in the opening position. Breathe in deeply and raise your arms above your head.

2 As you breathe out, lower your arms and visualize stagnant qi being drawn out of your body, through the soles of your feet, deep into the

PLANT THERAPY

Looking at green plants helps to reduce blood pressure and anxiety during stressful activities. Relaxing in a room with a view of a tree produces a more rapid reduction in blood pressure than relaxing in a viewless room.

earth. As it drains away, imagine fresh qi coming in through the top of your head. Feel tension and fatigue drain away as your qi is recharged.

3 Visualize the fresh qi flowing through your body, then settling just below your navel (in an area called the tan tien; see page 62). With practice, you might start to feel a vibration and warmth in this area as qi becomes concentrated there.

FLOATATION THERAPY

Today, I'd like you to book a series of at least four floatations at your nearest float center. Floatation therapy can help you achieve the deepest relaxation possible without falling asleep, and a single float lasting 45 minutes has been shown to lower hypertension. You lie in a lightproof, sound-insulated tank containing a shallow pool of water at body temperature, to which Epsom salts (magnesium sulfate) is added. This forms a super-saturated solution of saline even more buoyant than the Dead Sea. Floating frees your brain from its usual sensory distractions; as a result, your brain more easily generates theta waves, which are associated with feelings of calm.

DAY FOURTEEN

DAILY MENU

Breakfast: homemade muesli (see page 141) with pomegranate and blueberries
Morning snack: a piece of fruit
Lunch: baked sweet potato. Low-fat cottage cheese. Arugula. Bean sprouts with grated beet, celery, and walnuts. Low-fat yogurt with live cultures with fresh fruit
Afternoon snack: a handful of walnuts
Dinner: sea bass with lime and cilantro (see page 188). Broccoli. Couscous. Walnut and fruit compote (see page 195)

Drinks: 2½ cups 2% or 1% milk. Freshly squeezed fruit/veg juice. Unlimited green, black, white, or herbal tea, and mineral water. 5 ounces (⅔ cup) red wine or unsweetened red grape juice
Supplements: see page 158

DAILY EXERCISE ROUTINE

Today, and from now on, walk briskly for 45 minutes or cycle for 30 minutes on most days of the week. Also do your muscle-toning exercises from days one through seven. In the evening, wind down with the qigong sequence. Today's exercise, in which you redirect qi to the tan tien, completes the sequence.

QIGONG—CLOSING EXERCISE

1 Stand in the opening position. Let your body sink a little at your knees and waist. Bring your hands to the front of your body, at the level of your navel, palms facing upward and the tips of your fingers almost touching.
2 Breathe in and raise qi by straightening your body and gently curving your arms up until your palms face your forehead.
3 Breathe out and turn your palms downward—push them down as far as they will go, then let your arms relax.
4 Repeat this raising and lowering six times. Then bring your hands to rest on top of each other over your tan tien. Visualize qi energy flowing out of your hands into your navel area. After a minute or two, return to the opening position.

CONSULTING A REFLEXOLOGIST

Today, I suggest a consultation with a reflexologist. Reflexology works on reflex points on your feet. Having asked you about your medical history, as well as your current health and lifestyle, a reflexologist will ask you to remove your footwear and relax on a seat or couch with your feet raised. He or she will apply a light dusting of talcum powder to their hands, then use their fingers and thumbs to stimulate reflex points all over your feet. The aim is to find any points of tenderness and then massage these points to break up deposits under the skin. This promotes energy flow and opens up blocked nerve pathways. Your treatment will then focus on areas of the foot associated with high blood pressure (see page 53). A session usually lasts 45 to 60 minutes. Afterward, you should feel a profound sense of relaxation. To find a reflexologist, see page 237.

CONTINUING THE MODERATE PROGRAM

Well done! You have followed the moderate program for two weeks. Now I would like you to continue with the eating plan for two more weeks. This will give you an entire month of healthy eating and make you very well-acquainted with the foods you need to buy and eat. After this point you can start to vary the foods you eat, and include some new recipes. The following information will enable you to plan your long-term future using the moderate program principles.

YOUR LONG-TERM DIET

The diet you have been following is an advanced, lower glycemic index diet that, as well as following the basic principles of the DASH diet (see page 66), also includes extra foods that are beneficial for people with hypertension. These superfoods (see pages 80–86) have a significant blood pressure-lowering effect. These guidelines will help you continue on this diet:

- Eat as many superfoods, such as almonds, apples, oats, oily fish, and pumpkin seeds, as you can every day (see pages 80–86 for a full list).
- Continue to use the low-glycemic index grains included in the moderate plan, such as hemp pasta, red rice, wild rice, and quinoa.
- Every week, have two or three vegetarian days, eat fish two or three times, and meat only once or twice.
- Sprout a variety of beans and seeds at home.
- Keep making your own combinations of fruit and vegetable juices, and fresh herbal teas.

RECIPES

Explore fish-based and vegetarian recipes—you will find more at www.naturalhealthguru.co.uk, and you can post your favorites there for other followers of the moderate program to try. You don't have to follow formal recipes on the moderate program: simply broiling or baking fish with olive oil, lemon or lime juice, fresh herbs, and black pepper provides a delicious, quick and healthy meal. Team this with lightly steamed fresh vegetables or a salad, plus a low-glycemic index grain, and you have a meal that is beneficial to the health of your cardiovascular system.

SELECTING FISH

Because fish will play a prominent part in your long-term diet it's useful to know how to select fish that is in optimum condition—and also how much to buy. Here are some guidelines:

- Inspect the fish—its skin should gleam like finest shot silk. It should smell of seawater—salty, with a tang of ozone, rather than smelling fishy. A fishy smell is the result of chemical breakdown that suggests the fish is not optimally fresh. The eyes of the fish should be clear, bright, and shiny; the gills should be a healthy pink or bright red; and the scales should be tight.
- Perform the "prod test"—poke the flesh with your finger. It should feel moist and firm to the touch, and spring back with elasticity, rather than remain collapsed. This test is useful even if the fish is ultra-fresh—even fresh fish can be flabby and in poor condition.
- Pick up shellfish to assess their weight—they should always seem heavy for their size. Make sure bivalve molluscs, such as mussels, shut firmly on tapping and are not coated with decaying weeds, barnacles, or mud. Discard any that do not close, or any cooked ones that are not open.
- Wastage with fish varies from around one-third with monkfish to more than two-thirds with lobster. As a general rule, buy double or triple the amount you want to eat. Don't discard bones—simmer them up with herbs and vegetables to make fish stock.

YOUR LONG-TERM SUPPLEMENT REGIME

Continue taking the recommended supplements for the moderate program (see page 158) long term. If you have taken only the supplements on the recommended list, you might wish to add in one or more of the supplements in the optional list for extra benefit. Full details of each

SLEEP QUALITY

Pay attention to the quality of your sleep. Poor sleep is both a source of and a cause of stress. Follow these basic sleep guidelines: go to bed at the same time each night; avoid anything that is stimulating or stressful in the evenings (for example, caffeine, a large meal, exercise, or work); make sure your bedroom is dark and peaceful; and get sufficient exercise and natural light during the day.

supplement, including updates on latest research findings, are available at www.naturalhealthguru.co.uk

YOUR EXERCISE ROUTINE

After two weeks of doing the muscle-toning exercises, you should have started to notice a difference in your muscle tone. Continue these exercises and, if you do not yet belong to a gym, consider joining one and having a session with a personal trainer. Aim to do at least 45 minutes of aerobic exercise on most days and continue to unwind with the qigong exercises at the end of the day.

YOUR THERAPY PROGRAM

Continue to meditate at least once a day for 20 minutes, or, ideally, once in the morning and once in the evening. Also continue doing any of the breathing exercises as these can intensify the power of your meditation. If you find it helpful, visit a medical herbalist and/or a reflexologist on a regular basis. Consider booking regular float sessions at a floatation centre if you found the experience relaxing.

MONITORING YOUR BLOOD PRESSURE

While continuing with the moderate program, monitor your blood pressure on a weekly basis, at the same time of day, unless your doctor has asked you to check it more frequently. Record your blood pressure measurements in a chart (use a copy of the one on page 112), so you have an easily accessible record.

If your blood pressure is consistently below 130/80 mmHg, well done. The moderate program suits you, and you should continue it long term. If you're taking anti–hypertensive medication, your doctor might consider reducing this, if he or she judges that it's appropriate. This is not something you should do without your doctor's supervision as certain anti–hypertensive drugs need to be reduced slowly.

If your blood pressure is consistently between 130/80 mmHg and 140/90 mmHg, consider moving up to the full-strength program to see if you can bring it down to below 130/80 mmHg.

If your blood pressure is consistently above 140/90 mmHg, you can move onto the full-strength program, but you should also consult your doctor before you do so.

BREAKFAST RECIPES

VANILLA ROOIBOS COMPOTE
SERVES 4

1 vanilla rooibos herbal teabag
1¼ cups boiling water
8 slices dried apple
8 dried apricots
8 dried figs
8 dried prunes
1 handful raisins
Low-fat fromage blanc or yogurt with
   live cultures, to serve
1 handful slivered almonds, walnut
   halves, or mixed seeds, to serve
   (optional)

1 Put the teabag in a heatproof bowl,
   pour the water over, and leave until
   cool; remove the teabag.

2 Put the fruit in a bowl, pour the tea
   over, and refrigerate overnight. Top
   with fromage blanc or yogurt, and
   nuts or seeds.

SPICY GARLIC MUSHROOMS
SERVES 4

shallots, sliced
2 scallions, sliced
2-inch piece gingerroot, peeled and
   grated
2 garlic cloves, crushed
1 fresh red chili, seeded and sliced
5 cups halved button mushrooms
1 tablespoon olive oil
⅔ cup dry white wine
1 handful fresh cilantro or flat-leaf
   parsley, roughly chopped
4 slices wholewheat toast, to serve
Freshly ground black pepper

1 Fry the shallots, scallions, ginger,
   garlic, chili, and mushrooms in the oil.

2 Add the white wine and simmer
   gently. Season and stir in the herbs.
   Serve hot on toast.

FIGS WITH POMEGRANATE

SERVES 4

1 pomegranate
8 fresh figs
½ cup low-fat fromage blanc

1 Slice the crown end off the pomegranate and score the rind from top to bottom in six places around the fruit. Put the pomegranate in a bowl of water and break the sections apart. Tear away the thin membranes and pry out the seeds. The seeds will sink, while the bitter-tasting membranes and skin will float for easy separation; drain, reserving the seeds.

2 Make two deep cuts in the top of each fig to form a cross. Gently open out the figs, so each one forms a tuliplike shape. Mix the fromage blanc with the pomegranate seeds, saving a few seeds to serve.

3 Put the figs on a serving plate. Spoon the fromage blanc mixture into the figs and serve any remaining on the side. Sprinkle with the reserved pomegranate seeds and serve.

RASPBERRY AND BRAZIL NUT MEDLEY

SERVES 4

3¼ cups raspberries
2 cups silken tofu, roughly cut into chunks
⅔ cup roughly chopped Brazil nuts

1 Set 2 tablespoons of raspberries aside for serving. Put the remaining raspberries in a blender with the tofu and process until smooth. Divide the mixture between four glass serving bowls.

2 Sprinkle the chopped brazil nuts over each serving, top with the reserved raspberries, and serve.

LUNCH RECIPES

BLACK BEAN COMPOTE WITH CUMIN AND CILANTRO

SERVES 4

1¼ cups dried black beans, soaked
  overnight
1½ teaspoons extra virgin olive oil
1 large red onion, chopped
1 large green bell pepper, chopped
2 garlic cloves, crushed
1 teaspoon cumin seeds, freshly ground
4 tomatoes, skinned, seeded, and
  chopped
1 handful fresh cilantro leaves, roughly
  chopped
Freshly squeezed juice of 1 lime
Freshly ground black pepper
Crusty whole-wheat bread, to serve

1 Drain and rinse the beans, put in a
   pan, cover with water and bring to
   a boil. Simmer 1 to 1½ hours until
   tender; then drain.

2 Heat the oil in a pan. Add the onion,
   green pepper, garlic, and cumin, and
   stir-fry 5 minutes. Add the tomatoes
   and beans and almost cover with cold
   water. Bring to a boil, then simmer
   10 minutes.

3 Stir in the cilantro leaves and lime
   juice. Season with black pepper and
   serve with bread.

CREAM OF WATERCRESS SOUP

SERVES 4

2 potatoes, peeled and roughly chopped
1 onion, chopped
2 garlic cloves, crushed
1 quart vegetable stock (see page 153)
  or water
1 large bunch watercress, roughly
  chopped
⅔ cup low-fat fromage blanc
Freshly grated nutmeg
Freshly ground black pepper

1 Put the potatoes, onion, garlic, and
   stock in a large saucepan. Bring to
   a boil, lower the heat, and leave to
   simmer gently 15 minutes.

2 Add the watercress to the pan and
   cook 5 minutes longer. Leave to
   cool slightly, then purée in a blender,
   in batches, if necessary. Stir in the
   fromage blanc, then season to taste
   with nutmeg or black pepper. Serve
   hot or cold.

WARM CHICKPEA SALAD

SERVES 4

1½ teaspoons extra virgin olive oil
1 red onion, chopped
2 garlic cloves, crushed
1 red bell pepper, roughly chopped
1 can (15-oz.) chickpeas, drained
1 large tomato, skinned, seeded, and
  chopped
Freshly squeezed juice of 1 lemon
1 handful bean sprouts
1 handful fresh parsley or dill, roughly
  chopped
Freshly ground black pepper
Wholewheat pita bread, to serve

1 Heat the oil in a large pan. Add the
   onion, garlic, and red pepper and
   cook over medium heat until soft.
   Stir in the chickpeas and cook until
   hot and starting to color.

2 Add the tomato and lemon juice and
   cook 2 minutes. Add the bean sprouts
   and stir over low heat until warm. Stir
   in the parsley or dill and season with
   black pepper. Serve with warm pita
   bread.

SMOKED MACKEREL AND MANGO MEDLEY

SERVES 4

9 ounces mixed baby salad leaves
4 peppered, smoked mackerel fillets,
  skinned and chopped into bite-size
  pieces
1 large, ripe mango, peeled, pitted, and
  flesh cubed
1 ripe avocado, peeled, pitted, and flesh
  cubed
4 scallions, chopped
1 handful bean sprouts
1 handful fresh cilantro leaves
Freshly squeezed juice of 1 lime
2 tablespoons extra virgin olive oil or
  walnut oil
1 teaspoon honey

1 Put the salad leaves in a serving bowl.
   Carefully mix together the mackerel,
   mango, avocado, scallions, bean
   sprouts, and cilantro leaves in another
   bowl and set aside.

2 Put the lime juice, oil, and honey in
   a screw-top jar and shake vigorously.
   Pour over the mackerel and mango
   mixture and toss to mix through.
   Tip the mackerel mixture over the
   salad leaves and serve.

DINNER RECIPES

SOUSED HERRINGS

SERVES 4

For the marinade:
1¼ cups red wine vinegar
2 juniper berries
2 cloves
1 bay leaf
3 black peppercorns, crushed

4 large herrings, gutted and cleaned,
   with heads and backbones removed
4 teaspoons wholegrain mustard
4 shallots, thinly sliced
Rye bread, to serve

1 Heat the oven to 350°F.

2 Put the marinade ingredients in a
   pan and gently bring to a boil. Lower
   the heat and simmer 10 minutes.
   Set aside to cool a little, then strain,
   discarding the spices and bay leaf.

3 Open each herring and spread
   with mustard. Set 1 tablespoon of
   the shallots aside and arrange the
   remainder in a row down the middle
   of each fish. Roll up from head to tail
   and secure with a wooden toothpick.

4 Put the herrings in a baking dish and
   pour the strained marinade over.
   Sprinkle with the reserved shallots,
   cover, and bake 15 minutes. Leave
   to cool. Leave to souse in the
   refrigerator for at least 2 days. Serve
   with rye bread.

ROAST TOMATO AND RED PEPPER SOUP

SERVES 4

8 ripe tomatoes, cut in half
4 large red bell peppers, cut in half and
   seeded
4 garlic cloves
1½ teaspoons olive oil, plus extra for
   drizzling
1 onion, chopped
2½ cups vegetable stock (see page 153)
   or water
Freshly squeezed juice of 1 lemon
Freshly ground black pepper
1 handful fresh flat-leaf parsley, roughly
   chopped, to serve

1 Heat the oven to 375°F.

2 Put the tomatoes cut-side up on a
   baking sheet, together with the red
   pepper and garlic. Drizzle with oil
   and bake 30 minutes.

3 Heat 1½ teaspoons oil in a pan.
   Add the onion and cook until soft.
   Add the tomatoes, red peppers,
   garlic, and stock. Bring to a boil,
   then simmer 15 minutes. Leave to
   cool a little, then purée in a blender.

4 Return to the pan and heat through.
   Stir in the lemon juice, season with
   black pepper, and serve sprinkled
   with parsley.

FRENCH ONION SOUP

SERVES 4

2 tablespoons olive oil
4 large onions, thinly sliced
2 garlic cloves, crushed
1 quart vegetable stock (see page 153)
   or water
1 sprig rosemary
1 sprig thyme
1 bay leaf
Freshly ground black pepper
1 handful fresh flat-leaf parsley, roughly
   chopped, to serve

1 Heat the oil in a large saucepan.
   Add the onions and garlic and cook
   over medium-high heat until they
   start to color.

2 Pour in the stock, rosemary, thyme,
   and bay leaf. Bring to a boil, lower the
   heat, and leave to simmer 30 minutes.
   Remove the herbs, season to taste
   with black pepper, and serve
   sprinkled with parsley.

SEA BASS WITH LIME AND CILANTRO

SERVES 4

4 sea bass fillets, about 7 ounces each
Freshly squeezed juice of 2 limes
2 tablespoons olive oil
2 garlic cloves, crushed
1 handful fresh cilantro leaves, roughly
   chopped
1 lime, sliced, to serve

1 Put the sea bass fillets in a single
   layer in a shallow, baking dish. Mix
   together the lime juice, oil, garlic, and
   cilantro leaves and pour over the fish.
   Leave to marinate in the refrigerator
   at least 30 minutes. Meanwhile, heat
   the broiler to medium-hot.

2 Broil the fish in the dish 10 minutes
   until the flesh is just firm. Baste the
   fish frequently with the lime and
   cilantro marinade while broiling.
   Serve with the lime slices on the side.

CINNAMON EGGPLANTS

SERVES 4

2 large eggplants
2 tablespoons olive oil
2 large onions
4 garlic cloves
2 large tomatoes, skinned, seeded,
   and chopped
½ teaspoon acacia honey
12 fresh basil leaves, torn
½ teaspoon ground cinnamon
Grated peel and freshly squeezed juice
   of 1 unwaxed lemon
1 handful chopped almonds
Freshly ground black pepper

1 Heat the oven to 350°F.

2 Put the eggplants in a large pan and cover with boiling water. Return to a boil and cook 10 minutes; drain, then plunge into cold water to cool. Cut each eggplant in half lengthwise. Scoop out and reserve most of the flesh, leaving a ½-inch thick shell. Lightly oil the insides of the eggplant shells and season with black pepper. Put on a greased baking sheet and bake 30 minutes.

3 Meanwhile, chop the eggplant flesh and set aside. Heat the remaining oil in a skillet, add the onion and garlic, and cook about 5 minutes until soft. Add the tomatoes, honey, basil, and cinnamon and leave to simmer 15 minutes. Add the eggplant flesh, lemon juice and peel, and almonds. Cook 10 minutes longer; season with black pepper.

4 Remove the eggplant shells from the oven, fill with the hot tomato and eggplant mixture, and serve.

STUFFED VINE LEAVES WITH TZATZIKI

SERVES 4

20 grape leaves, fresh or canned

1½ teaspoons olive oil

3 shallots, finely chopped

4 garlic cloves, crushed

heaped ½ cup brown rice, rinsed and drained

3 tablespoons golden raisins

3 tablespoons slivered almonds

Grated peel and freshly squeezed juice of 1 unwaxed lemon

3½ cups vegetable stock (see page 153) or water

6 scallions, finely chopped

1 handful fresh mint leaves, roughly chopped

1 handful fresh flat-leaf parsley, roughly chopped

Freshly ground black pepper

For the tzatziki:

1 cucumber, peeled and coarsely grated

¾ cup low-fat yogurt with live cultures

2 garlic cloves, crushed

1 handful fresh mint leaves, finely chopped

Grated peel and freshly squeezed juice of 1 unwaxed lemon

1 If using fresh grape leaves, plunge them into boiling water 1 minute, drain, and remove the coarse stems. If using canned leaves, rinse them under cold running water.

2 Heat the oil in a large pan. Add the shallots and garlic and fry about 5 minutes. Add the rice, golden raisins, almonds, and lemon peel and cook 1 minute. Add enough stock to cover the rice and cook until the rice is tender. Leave to cool, then stir in the scallions, mint, and parsley; season with pepper.

3 Put a spoonful of the rice mixture on each grape leaf and fold the leaf around it to make a bundle. Pack the bundles tightly in a pan. Cover with stock and sprinkle with the lemon juice. Put a plate on top of the bundles to keep them submerged. Cover with a lid or foil and simmer over very low heat 50 minutes.

4 Make the tzatziki by mixing all the ingredients together. Season with black pepper. Serve the stuffed grape leaves with the tzatziki as a dip.

ROASTED RED PEPPERS
WITH HERBY BULGUR WHEAT

SERVES 4

2 large red bell peppers, cut in half lengthwise, cored, and seeded (stems intact)

2 large orange bell peppers, cut in half lengthwise, cored, and seeded (stems intact)

2 tablespoons olive oil

16 cherry tomatoes, cut in half

½ cup low-fat fromage blanc

4 tablespoons pesto

2 garlic cloves, crushed

2 tablespoons pine nuts

Freshly ground black pepper

For the herby bulgur wheat:

Heaped ½ cup bulgur wheat

3 cups vegetable stock (see page 153) or water

Grated peel and freshly squeezed juice of 1 unwaxed lemon

1 small handful fresh cilantro leaves, finely chopped

1 small handful fresh mint leaves, finely chopped

1 small handful fresh flat-leaf parsley, finely chopped

12 fresh basil leaves, torn

4 scallions, finely chopped

1 Heat the oven to 350°F.

2 Put the peppers cut-side up on a baking sheet and lightly brush with oil. Put 4 tomato halves in each pepper half.

3 Mash together the fromage blanc, pesto, and garlic and spoon over the tomatoes in each pepper half. Season to taste with black pepper and sprinkle over the pine nuts. Drizzle with a little more oil and roast in the oven 45 minutes, until the pepper skins start to char.

4 Meanwhile, put the bulgur wheat and stock in a large pan and bring to a boil. Lower the heat and simmer gently about 10 minutes, until all the liquid is absorbed. Stir in the lemon juice and peel, herbs, and scallions. Serve one red and one orange pepper half per person with a side helping of herby bulgur wheat.

STIR-FRIED TURKEY
WITH BEAN SPROUTS
SERVES 4

For the marinade:

2 tablespoons low-sodium soy sauce

1 tablespoon dry sherry

1 tablespoon olive oil

1 tablespoon honey

Freshly squeezed juice of 1 orange

2 garlic cloves, crushed

2-inch piece gingerroot, peeled and
   grated

4 skinless turkey breast halves, about
   7 ounces

3 tablespoons olive oil or unrefined
   virgin coconut oil

4 scallions, chopped

1 handful bean sprouts

2 cups shredded white cabbage

1 handful green beans, trimmed

1 tablespoon toasted sesame seeds

Freshly ground black pepper

1 Put all the marinade ingredients in a screw-top jar and shake vigorously to mix well. Lay the turkey in a shallow flameproof dish and pour half the marinade over. Turn the turkey breasts to coat them and leave to marinate at least 30 minutes. Heat the broiler to medium-hot.

2 Broil the turkey in the dish 10–15 minutes. Turn the meat halfway through cooking. Heat the oil in a large skillet. Add the scallions, bean sprouts, cabbage, and green beans and stir-fry 3 minutes. Pour in the remaining marinade and stir-fry 2 minutes longer.

3 Divide the stir-fry between 4 serving plates. Place a broiled turkey breast on top of each portion and sprinkle the sesame seeds over. Season with black pepper and serve.

MUSHROOM AND WALNUT LASAGNE

SERVES 4

1 tablespoon olive oil

1¾ cups chopped onions

1¾ cups chopped carrots

4 garlic cloves

6 celery stalks, chopped

1 handful mixed fresh herbs, such as thyme, parsley, oregano, and rosemary, roughly chopped

3 ripe tomatoes, skinned, seeded, and chopped, plus 1 tomato, thinly sliced

4¼ cups sliced mushrooms

1 handful walnut pieces

Freshly ground black pepper

12 sheets no-precook spinach or wholewheat lasagne sheets

1 cup low-fat fromage blanc

1¾ cups grated mozzarella cheese

1 Heat the oven to 350°F.

2 Heat the oil in a large skillet. Add the onions, carrots, garlic, celery, and herbs and fry over medium heat 10 minutes. Stir in the chopped tomatoes, mushrooms, and walnut pieces and cook 10 minutes longer. Season with black pepper.

3 Spread one third of the mushroom and walnut mixture over the base of a baking dish. Cover with 3 lasagne sheets, then spread these with one-third of the fromage blanc. Repeat these layers twice more. Top with the cheese and sliced tomato. Bake 45 minutes and serve.

ROSÉ TROUT

SERVES 4

4 trout fillets, about 6 ounces each

2 shallots, sliced into rings

1½ cups rosé wine

1 handful slivered almonds

Freshly ground black pepper

1 handful fresh dill, roughly chopped, to serve

1 Heat the oven to 350°F.

2 Put the trout fillets in a single layer in a baking dish. Sprinkle the shallots over the top and pour the wine over. Scatter the almonds over, cover, and bake about 30 minutes, or until the fillets are tender and flake easily. Serve immediately, sprinkled with the dill.

DESSERT RECIPES

BROILED MUSHROOMS WITH ALMONDS AND BASIL
SERVES 4

4 tablespoons olive oil
2 garlic cloves
2 scallions, chopped
1 handful slivered almonds
1 handful mixed seeds, such as pumpkin, sunflower, and sesame
4 large, flat mushrooms
1 handful wholewheat breadcrumbs
1 handful fresh basil leaves, roughly chopped
Freshly ground black pepper

1 Heat the oven to 350°F.

2 Heat the oil in a skillet. Add the garlic and scallions and cook over medium heat about 4 minutes until soft. Add the slivered almonds and mixed seeds and cook 1 minute longer, stirring.

3 Put the mushrooms hollow-side up in a shallow baking dish. Spoon the almond and seed mixture into the mushrooms. Sprinkle the breadcrumbs and basil over and season with black pepper. Cover with foil and bake 15 minutes. Serve immediately.

OAT FLUMMERY
SERVES 4

2 handfuls steel-cut oats
1 handful blanched almonds, roughly chopped
1 handful walnuts, roughly chopped
9 ounces silken tofu
2 ripe bananas, peeled and sliced
Grated peel and freshly squeezed juice of 1 unwaxed lemon
1 tablespoon honey (optional)

1 Lightly toast the oats and nuts under the broiler. Leave to cool.

2 Mash together the other ingredients, then chill them. Fold in the oats and nuts and serve.

MULLED FRUIT SALAD
SERVES 4

4 ripe peaches, cut in half, pitted, and sliced
8 fresh apricots, cut in half and pitted (or 8 dried, ready-to-eat apricots)
⅔ cup freshly squeezed orange juice
⅔ cup light red wine, such as Beaujolais
½ teaspoon ground cinnamon
1 handful raisins
2 bananas, peeled and thickly sliced

1 Simmer all the ingredients in a pan 10 minutes.

2 Serve warm.

BITES, SNACKS AND DRINKS

CREAMY TURKISH DELIGHT FIGS
SERVES 4

9 ounces silken tofu
Grated peel and freshly squeezed juice
   of 1 unwaxed orange
1 tablespoon honey
12 ripe fresh figs
1 to 2 tablespoons rosewater, for
   drizzling

1 Blend the tofu, orange juice, and
   honey in a blender.
2 Cut a cross in the top of each fig.
   Spoon the tofu into the figs. Sprinkle
   with orange peel and drizzle with
   rosewater.

WALNUT AND FRUIT COMPOTE
SERVES 4

1 small, ripe Galia melon, seeded and
   flesh divided into balls
1 red grapefruit, divided into segments
1 large banana, peeled and sliced
⅔ cup unsweetened apple juice
1 handful walnuts, roughly chopped

1 Halve each grapefruit segment
   lengthwise; remove and discard the
   outer membranes.
2 Put all the fruit in a bowl. Add the
   apple juice and walnuts and serve.

TOASTED MIXED NUTS
SERVES 4

1 handful blanched almonds
1 handful hazelnuts
1 handful unsalted cashew nuts
1 handful walnuts
1 handful Brazil nuts
1 handful raisins (optional)

1 Warm a large skillet over medium
   heat. Toast the nuts gently, moving
   and shaking the pan as they turn
   golden; take care not to burn them.
2 Let the nuts cool. Mix with the
   raisins, if using, and serve.

CHICKPEA AND AVOCADO HUMMUS
SERVES 4

1 can (15 oz.) chickpeas, drained
1 large ripe avocado
2 garlic cloves, crushed
Freshly squeezed juice of 1 lemon
Freshly ground black pepper
1 handful fresh mint leaves
Rice cakes, to serve

1 Put all the ingredients in a blender,
   except the rice cakes, and process
   until smooth.
2 Serve with rice cakes.

MOCK CAVIAR

SERVES 4

2 eggplants, cut in half lengthwise
2 scallions, finely chopped
2 garlic cloves, crushed
Freshly squeezed juice of 1 lemon
12 fresh basil leaves
4 tablespoons extra virgin olive oil
Freshly ground black pepper

1 Heat the oven to 400°F.

2 Put the eggplants cut-side down on a baking sheet. Bake 30 minutes. Leave to cool slightly, then scoop out the pulp into a bowl and discard the skin.

3 Place the eggplant pulp in a blender with the scallions, garlic, lemon juice, basil leaves, and oil; process until smooth and well blended. Season with black pepper and serve.

BERRY SMOOTHIE

SERVES 4

4 handfuls mixed berries, such as blackberries, raspberries, strawberries, and blueberries
2½ cups low-fat yogurt with live cultures or fromage blanc
1 tablespoon mixed seeds, such as pumpkin, sunflower, and sesame
2 tablespoons crushed ice
A little honey (optional)

1 Blend all the ingredients in a blender until smooth. If you wish, sweeten with a little honey.

2 Pour into tall glasses and serve.

INTRODUCING THE FULL-STRENGTH PROGRAM

The full-strength program is designed to bring your blood pressure down as efficiently as possible. It's ideal for people who have completed the moderate program; and for those who want to obtain the maximum beneficial effects for their hypertension and the health of their cardiovascular system. You need to be fit and healthy, and already eat a well-balanced diet with plenty of fresh fruit and vegetables.

There are 14 daily plans that you can repeat to create a 28-day program. Follow the full-strength program for at least a month before assessing its benefits. Once you feel comfortable with the diet and lifestyle changes involved, feel free to make your own adjustments.

THE FULL-STRENGTH PROGRAM DIET

The diet incorporates foods identified as having the most beneficial influence on the risk of heart attack and stroke, and which have the potential to increase life expectancy by six and a half years for men, and almost five years for women if eaten on a regular basis. The diet includes a high intake of almonds, garlic, dark chocolate, fruit and vegetables, plus fish three to four times a week. These superfoods were selected on the basis of evidence pooled from a number of scientific trials. Although the foods are similar to those found in the gentle and moderate programs, they are consumed with higher frequency.

If you are hypertensive but not on anti-hypertensive medication, you can expect to reduce your blood pressure by at least 9/4 mmHg on this program. And if you also take the recommended supplements, you may be able to lower your blood pressure by 15/8 mmHg or more over the course of one month. If you are taking anti-hypertensive drugs, the full-strength diet and supplement program will improve their effectiveness. It will also lower your total and LDL–cholesterol levels and reduce your triglyceride levels (see pages 72–73).

As I recommended in the other programs, dispose of any foods in your home that are high in sugar, salt, saturated fat and trans fats. Do not add salt during cooking or at the table. Obtain flavor from fresh herbs and black pepper instead. If you haven't yet started to make your own fruit and vegetable juices at home (see page 156), now is the time to start.

INCLUDING CHOCOLATE AND WINE IN YOUR DIET

Dark chocolate (at least 70 percent cocoa solids) contains powerful antioxidant polyphenols similar to those found in red wine and green tea, and the evidence for their positive effect on hypertension is strong.

Of all the superfoods, red wine has the most blood pressure-lowering benefits—but only when drunk in moderation. More than 5 ounces a day can have a harmful effect on health. Scientists have found that the highest content of beneficial antioxidants is found in wine made from Cabernet Sauvignon grapes. And, compared with red wines from other parts of the world, researchers from Glasgow University found that Cabernet Sauvignons from Chile have the highest amount of heart-friendly antioxidant flavonols. Narrowing things down even further, they found that Cabernet Sauvignons from the Viña MontGras estate have significantly more antioxidants than any other Chilean wine tested.

SHOPPING LIST

You will need all the food and drink items on the shopping list for the gentle program (see page 114). In addition, you will need the following (where possible, buy regularly in small quantities for optimum freshness).

DAIRY AND SOY PRODUCTS
buffalo mozzarella cheese, firm tofu, silken tofu

FRUIT AND VEGETABLES
blueberries, butternut squash or pumpkin, cooking apples, dried cranberries, guava, raspberries, strawberries

HERBS AND SPICES
dill, fennel seeds, green peppercorns, lemongrass

GRAINS
barley bread, hemp or spinach tagliatelle, lasagne or spaghetti, red rice, soy bread steel-cut oats, wild rice

PROTEINS
chickpeas, green lentils, herrings, lean pork fillets, lima beans, sea bass

MISCELLANEOUS
coconut milk

THE FULL-STRENGTH PROGRAM EXERCISE ROUTINE

The full-strength exercise program is designed for those who are relatively fit and who already exercise regularly for 45 minutes on most days. During the program, I recommend you increase the level of exercise you take to 45 to 60 minutes a day on at least five days a week. Try to find new forms of exercise so you build variety into your exercise program—that way you won't get bored. Perform stretching and weight exercises on the other two days so you're exercising most days or every day. As well as brisk walking, cycling, and swimming, consider bowling, golf, and similar activities that improve your social life as well as your health. Here are some other ways to be active:

- Walk rather than drive your children to school and then gently jog home.
- Walk everywhere—indoors as well as outdoors—at a brisk pace.
- Do manual chores (such as housework) as vigorously as possible.
- Reduce time spent on sedentary activities, such as watching television, and instead go for a bike ride or walk with friends, family, or even a borrowed dog if you don't own one yourself.
- Use the stairs rather than an elevator or escalator.
- Walk part or all of the way to your destinations—get off the bus or train one stop earlier than normal.

If you miss a day's exercise due to illness or time constraints, don't feel you've failed (exercise routines are at risk of lapsing after an unexpected interruption). Rather than giving up, resolve to get back to exercising as quickly as possible—plan exactly what you're going to do and when and don't let your slot of exercise time get filled up with a different activity—even if the other activity seems more pressing.

Whenever you're exercising, always warm up and cool down and, if you're cycling outdoors, wear appropriate safety equipment. Always monitor your 10-second pulse rate (see pages 101–102) to insure you're not overexerting yourself. The exercise routines in the full-strength program are more intense than in the previous two programs, so if you're in any doubt about your fitness, or you have angina or a history of heart

FULL-STRENGTH PROGRAM SUPPLEMENTS

These are the supplements I recommend you take while you're following the full-strength program. You can buy them from drug stores, supermarkets, and whole-food stores. Read about these supplements and how they lower your blood pressure on pages 86–92.

Recommended daily supplements
- Vitamin C (2,000 mg)
- Vitamin E (800 i.u/536 mg)
- Lycopene carotenoid complex (15 mg)
- Selenium (200 mcg)
- Coenzyme Q10 (120 mg)
- Garlic tablets (allicin yield 1,000–1,500 mcg)
- Omega-3 fish oil (900 mg daily; for example, 3x1 g fish oil capsules, each supplying 180 mg eicosapentaenoic acid, EPA, plus 120 mg docosahexaenoic acid, DHA)

Optional daily supplements (these will provide additional health benefits)
- Alpha lipoic acid (300 mg). Can be combined with L-carnitine in a 1:1 ratio
- Magnesium (300 mg)
- Calcium (1,000 mg)
- Folic acid (1,000 mcg) plus vitamin B12 (50 mcg)
- Reishi (1,500 mg)
- Bilberry fruit extracts (180 mg; standardized to give 25 percent anthocyanins)
- Probiotics (fermented milk drinks, live yogurt, or supplements)

attack, ask your doctor for guidance on how much exercise you can do. Stop exercising at once if you feel unwell.

THE FULL-STRENGTH PROGRAM THERAPIES

The full-strength program includes relaxation techniques, such as transcendental meditation, and practitioner-led therapies, such as naturopathy and acupuncture. If you're new to meditation, you might find it's difficult to focus your mind at first. This is normal. In time, you will find that the discipline of meditation helps mental chatter to lessen.

You will need to book two appointments with therapists in advance —please look at days seven and fourteen of the program now.

THE FULL-STRENGTH PROGRAM
DAY ONE

DAILY MENU

Breakfast: stuffed tomatoes (see page 226)
Morning snack: a portion of superfood fruit (see pages 80–86), such as apple, blueberries, cherries, figs, grapes, kiwi, guava, mango, or pomegranate
Lunch: almond trout (see page 228). Bowl of mixed salad leaves

sprinkled with walnuts, pumpkin seeds, chopped garlic, walnut oil, and red wine vinegar.
Fresh fruit
Afternoon snack: a handful of almonds
Dinner: broiled salmon steak marinated in olive oil and lime juice. Broccoli. Brown rice.

About 1½ ounces dark chocolate
Drinks: 2½ cups 2% or 1% milk. Freshly squeezed fruit/veg juice. Unlimited green, black, white, or herbal tea, and mineral water. 5 ounces (⅔ cup) red wine or unsweetened red grape juice
Supplements: see page 200

Over the next 14 days, I introduce you to a series of yoga postures that form a sequence known as the sun salutation. Regular yoga practice can lower systolic blood pressure by 10–15 mmHg.

DAILY EXERCISE ROUTINE

When you get up in the morning do the first posture of the sun salutation (see below). Walk briskly for 30 to 45 minutes during the day. Alternatively, swim or cycle for 20 minutes. In the evening, unwind by lying in the corpse pose (see page 136) for 15 minutes.

SUN SALUTATION—1ST POSTURE

1 Stand tall and straight with your feet together. Bend your elbows and bring your palms together in front of your chest in a prayerlike position.
2 Relax in this position for one minute. As you breathe in and out, visualize the sun rising. Imagine its warmth and light radiating through your body.

MEDITATION

Daily meditation can lower average systolic blood pressure by at least 10 mmHg within 12 weeks. During the first week, I suggest you meditate

AVOID INVERSION

The yoga sequence in this program includes some head-down poses that are not recommended if your blood pressure is 160/100 mmHg or higher. If this applies to you, follow the gentle or moderate program until your blood pressure is lower.

once a day for 10 to 20 minutes, always before a meal, such as breakfast or dinner. Then build up to meditating twice a day.

GOING-INWARD MEDITATION

1 Start your first meditation session by sitting in a comfortable position near a nonticking clock or watch. Close your eyes. Breathe slowly and naturally and allow your mind to empty.
2 Over the next 10 minutes, direct your consciousness inward, deeper and deeper, to a place of utter calm and peace.
3 Open your eyes. Remain seated for at least a minute.

DAY TWO

DAILY MENU

Breakfast: homemade muesli (see page 141) topped with banana and coconut shavings
Morning snack: a portion of superfood fruit (see day one)
Lunch: beet and tofu medley (see page 228). Bowl of mixed salad leaves sprinkled with grated carrot, Brazil nuts, pumpkin seeds, and Mediterranean herb oil (see page 230)
Afternoon snack: a handful of almonds
Dinner: winter vegetable stew with rosemary (see page 232). Almond-chocolate cups (see page 234)
Drinks: 2½ cups 2% or 1% milk. Freshly squeezed fruit/veg juice. Unlimited green, black, white, or herbal tea, and mineral water. 5 ounces (⅔ cup) red wine or unsweetened red grape juice
Supplements: see page 200

DAILY EXERCISE ROUTINE

When you get up in the morning do the first posture of the sun salutation (see day one) followed by the next posture (see opposite). Walk briskly for 30 to 45 minutes during the day. Alternatively, swim or cycle for 20 minutes. In the evening, unwind by lying in the corpse pose (see page 136).

SUN SALUTATION—2ND POSTURE

1 As you inhale, raise your arms out to the sides and then up in a wide circle. Let your palms meet over your head and your fingers point up.

2 Let your chest open and expand as your arms lift. Press your palms firmly together and look up at them.

3 Keeping your feet flat on the floor, stretch your arms up above your head so you are as tall as possible. Slowly bend back as far as is comfortable. Hold your breath and stay in this position for a few seconds, letting your mind empty.

MEDITATION

As well as performing the basic meditation that you did yesterday, I'd now like you to focus on your breathing—this will enable you to get into a meditative state more quickly.

BREATH MEDITATION

1 Sit quietly and comfortably with your eyes closed. Breathe in slowly and deeply through your nose, and then out through your mouth.

2 Focus your attention on how cool the air feels when you inhale, and how warm it feels when you breathe out.

3 With each out-breath, imagine tension leaving your body. Feel yourself become more and more relaxed with each breath.

4 Start counting your breaths, saying the number of each breath as you let it go. This gives you something to focus on and helps to stop thoughts distracting you.

5 Now switch to breathing in through your mouth, and out through your nose. Decide which pattern of breathing feels most comfortable for you and continue this for the rest of today's meditation. Meditate for 10 to 20 minutes.

DAY THREE

DAILY MENU

Breakfast: herring in oats (see page 225). Broiled tomato. Wholewheat or rye toast
Morning snack: a portion of superfood fruit (see day one)
Lunch: bowl of mixed salad leaves sprinkled with sprouted beans, beet, carrot, red bell pepper, walnuts, pumpkin seeds, chopped garlic, walnut oil, and red wine vinegar. Wholewheat roll. Low-fat yogurt with live cultures with fresh fruit
Afternoon snack: a handful of almonds
Dinner: Mediterranean mackerel (see page 233). Wholewheat or hemp pasta. Broccoli. Baked apples (see page 235) with low-fat fromage blanc
Drinks: 2½ cups 2% or 1% milk. Freshly squeezed fruit/veg juice. Unlimited green, black, white, or herbal tea, and mineral water. 5 ounces (⅔ cup) red wine or unsweetened red grape juice
Supplements: see page 200

DAILY EXERCISE ROUTINE

When you get up in the morning do the first two postures of the sun salutation (see days one and two) followed by the posture below. Walk briskly for 30 to 45 minutes during the day. Alternatively, swim or cycle for 20 minutes. In the evening, unwind by lying in the corpse pose (see page 136) for 15 minutes.

SUN SALUTATION—3RD POSTURE

1 Breathe out and bend forward from your waist, keeping your arms straight out in front of you, and your palms together.
2 Bend as low as you can while keeping your back straight. Tuck your head in. Hold this position as long as feels comfortable, breathing in and out gently through your nose.

MEDITATION

Today, I'd like you to practice either of the meditations you have learned in the previous two days. But, beforehand, I'd like you to practice a yogic breathing exercise called sitkari (folded-up tongue). This technique "cools" the mind and helps you get into a meditative state more quickly.

SITKARI PRANAYAMA

1 Sit quietly and comfortably, with your back straight and your eyes closed. Start by breathing in, slowly and deeply, through your mouth, then out through both nostrils.

2 Fold your tongue back and gently press the tip of your tongue against the roof of your mouth. This leaves a narrow opening on either side of your tongue.

3 Inhale through these side openings—make a hissing sound with your breath. Continue to breathe out, slowly and deeply, through your nose. Repeat this several times.

4 When you are ready, return to normal, slow rhythmic breathing. Let your mind empty for your chosen meditation.

DAY FOUR

DAILY MENU

Breakfast: oatmeal with Brazil nuts and apricots
Morning snack: a portion of superfood fruit (see day one)
Lunch: almond and broccoli salad (see page 227) served with mixed salad leaves sprinkled with pumpkin seeds and Mediterranean herb oil (see page 230). Wholewheat roll. Low-fat yogurt with live cultures with fresh fruit
Afternoon snack: chocolate florentines (see page 236)
Dinner: lemon pork (see page 232). Spinach. Wholewheat or hemp pasta. About 1½ ounces dark chocolate
Drinks: 2½ cups 2% or 1% milk. Freshly squeezed fruit/veg juice. Unlimited green, black, white, or herbal tea, and mineral water. 5 ounces (⅔ cup) red wine or unsweetened red grape juice
Supplements: see page 200

Today you are going to meditate on a yantra, an ancient, geometric design that, because of its shape, is believed to act as a doorway to higher universal energies and bring you closer to enlightenment.

Yantra designs are many thousands of years old. Unlike other geometric designs used in meditation, such as mandalas, yantras are revealed to the world by a clairvoyant tantric guru—you cannot make one up. The chatter of the mind quickly ceases when you focus on a yantra during meditation.

DAILY EXERCISE ROUTINE

When you get up in the morning do the first three postures of the sun salutation (see days one through three) followed by the posture below. Walk briskly for 30 to 45 minutes or swim or cycle for 20 minutes during the day. In the evening, unwind in corpse pose (see page 136) for 15 minutes.

SUN SALUTATION—4TH POSTURE

1 From the third posture fold forward further to grasp the backs of your ankles or calves (or as far down your leg as you can).
2 Tuck your chin in and bend your elbows to pull your upper body gently in toward your legs.
3 Breathe out and hold your breath for a few seconds.

MEDITATION

Select a yantra to which you feel drawn (images and posters are available on the internet). Place the image so its middle is at eye level when you sit down.

YANTRA MEDITATION

1 Focus on the middle of the yantra. Now widen your area of focus so you can see the whole design.
2 When you feel ready, close your eyes and picture the yantra in your mind. Repeat these steps for 10 to 15 minutes.

MEDITATION POSTURES
Good postures for meditation include sitting upright in a straight-backed chair or sitting cross-legged on the floor with your hands resting in your lap or on your knees.

DAY FIVE

DAILY MENU

Breakfast: broiled tomatoes sprinkled with thyme. Wholewheat, rye, soy, or barley toast

Morning snack: a portion of superfood fruit (see day one)

Lunch: green minestrone (see page 227). Wholewheat roll. Low-fat yogurt with live cultures with fresh fruit

Afternoon snack: a handful of almonds

Dinner: mackerel and cucumber in wine (see page 232). Brown rice mixed with wild rice. Chocolate petit fours (see page 236)

Drinks: 2½ cups 2% or 1% milk. Freshly squeezed fruit/veg juice. Unlimited green, black, white, or herbal tea, and mineral water. 5 ounces (⅔ cup) red wine or unsweetened red grape juice

Supplements: see page 200

Today's dinner provides an excellent source of omega-3 fatty acids, selenium, and vitamins B3, B6, and B12 in the form of mackerel. Weight for weight, mackerel provides more omega-3 fatty acids than any other oily fish. Research shows that eating mackerel three times a week over an eight-month period significantly lowered both systolic and diastolic blood pressure in a group of people with essential hypertension.

DAILY EXERCISE ROUTINE

When you get up, do the first four postures of the sun salutation (see days one through four) followed by the posture below. Walk briskly for 30 to 45 minutes during the day. Alternatively, swim or cycle for 20 minutes. In the evening, unwind by lying in the corpse pose (see page 136) for 15 minutes.

SUN SALUTATION—5TH POSTURE

1 Following on from the fourth posture, breathe in, let go of your legs, and stand up straight.

2 As you breathe out, step forward as far as you can with your right leg, bend your right knee, and place both hands on the floor, arms straight, on each side of your right foot. As you come forward onto the ball of your left foot, keep your left knee off the floor.

3 Tilt your head back to look up. The next time you do this exercise, lunge forward with your left foot instead.

MEDITATION

Today I'd like you to select a personal mantra—a word or phrase to say to yourself as you breathe out. A mantra helps you reach a higher state of consciousness.

MANTRA MEDITATION

1 Choose a word that reflects your spiritual beliefs (for example, "Amen" or "Shalom"), a sound you are instinctively drawn to (for example, "om" or "aaaaaaah"), or a word you find helpful (for example, "calm").
2 Close your eyes and sit quietly, breathing in through your nose, and out through your mouth. Start whispering your mantra on each out-breath in a soft, rhythmic, and relaxed way. Do this for 10 to 15 minutes.

DAY SIX

DAILY MENU

Breakfast: blueberry and almond mousse (see page 225). Slice of wholegrain, rye, soy, or barley toast **Morning snack:** a portion of superfood fruit (see day one) **Lunch:** cheese, fruit, and nut platter (see page 229). Bowl of mixed salad leaves sprinkled with Brazil nuts, pumpkin seeds, chopped garlic, walnut oil, and red wine vinegar. Low-fat bio yogurt with live cultures **Afternoon snack:** a handful of almonds **Dinner:** chickpea curry (see page 231). Almond rice pudding (see page 234). About 1½ ounces dark chocolate **Drinks:** 2½ cups 2% or 1% milk. Freshly squeezed fruit/veg juice. Unlimited green, black, white, or herbal tea, and mineral water. 5 ounces (⅔ cup) red wine or unsweetened red grape juice **Supplements:** see page 200

DAILY EXERCISE ROUTINE

When you get up in the morning do the first five postures of the sun salutation (see days one through five) followed by the posture below. Walk briskly for 30 to 45 minutes or swim or cycle for 20 minutes during the day. In the evening, unwind by lying in the corpse pose (see page 136) for 15 minutes.

SUN SALUTATION—6TH POSTURE

1 From the fifth posture, straighten your upper body and gently move your arms out to the side and up.
2 Bring your palms together over your head, fingers pointing to the sky. Look up at your hands.
3 Hold your breath in this position for a few seconds. Keep your mind as empty as possible.

MEDITATION

Today you're going to meditate on the chakras—seven energy centers within your subtle body (see page 61).

CHAKRA MEDITATION

1 Start by meditating on the first chakra, the root chakra, by bringing your awareness to the base of your spine and visualizing the color red.
2 Move your awareness to your sacral chaka, at your sacrum, and imagine the color orange.
3 Move up to the next chakra, the solar plexus. Imagine a yellow color.
4 Focus on the middle of your chest, your heart chakra, and visualize the color green.
5 Move your awareness to your throat. Imagine sky blue.
6 Focus on the sixth chakra, the brow chakra, which sits between your eyes. Visualize indigo.
7 Finally, visualize the color violet at the top of your head, your crown chakra. Then imagine white light expanding from this chakra and enveloping you in a sphere of energy. Enjoy the feeling of calm and peace.

DAY SEVEN

DAILY MENU

Breakfast: Windward Islands trout (see page 225). Slice of wholegrain, rye, soy, or barley toast
Morning snack: a portion of superfood fruit (see day one)
Lunch: bowl of mixed salad leaves sprinkled with grated carrot, beet, bean sprouts, sliced button mushrooms, and Mediterranean herb oil (see page 230). Wholewheat roll. Low-fat yogurt with live cultures with fresh fruit
Afternoon snack: toasted almonds with seeds (see page 236)
Dinner: Oriental tofu stir-fry (see page 230). Red rice. A piece of fresh fruit
Drinks: 2½ cups 2% or 1% milk. Freshly squeezed fruit/veg juice. Unlimited green, black, white, or herbal tea, and mineral water. 5 ounces (⅔ cup) red wine or unsweetened red grape juice
Supplements: see page 200

DAILY EXERCISE ROUTINE

When you get up in the morning do the first six postures of the sun salutation (see days one through six) followed by the posture below. Walk briskly for 30 to 45 minutes or swim or cycle for 20 minutes. In the evening, unwind by lying in the corpse pose (see page 136) for 15 minutes.

SUN SALUTATION—7TH POSTURE

1 Following straight on from the last posture, breathe out and bring both hands down onto the floor on each side of your right foot.
2 Step back with your right foot so both feet are together. Straighten your body so you're in the straight-backed plank position (see page 168).
3 Hold this position for as long as is comfortable, breathing gently in and out, keeping your mind as quiet as possible.

SLOW BREATHING

If you feel stressed, make a conscious effort to slow down your breathing. Imagine a candle in front of your face. Exhale slowly—so that the candle just flickers slightly.

CONSULTING A NATUROPATH

Now you are halfway through the program, I suggest you see an accredited naturopath (see page 237). Many are trained in homeopathy, herbal medicine, chiropractic, and osteopathy, as well as nutritional medicine. During the first consultation, a naturopath will ask questions about your past and current health, and perform a medical examination that includes checking your blood pressure, listening to your heart and lungs, and, sometimes, examining your irises. He or she might also request blood tests, hair or sweat analyses (for mineral deficiencies), and x-rays. The naturopathic treatment of hypertension usually involves diet and lifestyle advice, breathing exercises, skin brushing (to boost circulation), nutritional supplements, herbal remedies, or homoeopathic medicines. You usually need at least four followup sessions of 30 minutes each.

DAY EIGHT

DAILY MENU

Breakfast: homemade muesli (see page 141) with raspberries and shaved coconut

Morning snack: a portion of superfood fruit (see day one)

Lunch: low-fat cottage cheese mixed with chopped pears and Brazil nuts. Bowl of mixed salad leaves sprinkled with pumpkin seeds and Mediterranean herb oil (see page 230). Wholewheat roll. Fresh fruit

Afternoon snack: a handful of almonds

Dinner: salmon steak marinated in olive oil, lime juice, and cilantro, then broiled. Arugula leaves and pumpkin seeds drizzled with walnut oil. Brown rice. About 1½ ounces dark chocolate

Drinks: 2½ cups 2% or 1% milk. Freshly squeezed fruit/veg juice. Unlimited green, black, white, or herbal tea, and mineral water. 5 ounces (⅔ cup) red wine or unsweetened red grape juice

Supplements: see page 200

From today I'd like you to meditate twice a day for 10 to 20 minutes each time. Start with 10 minutes twice a day and slowly build up to 15 or 20 minutes at each session. Choose whichever meditation you like for the second session.

DAILY EXERCISE ROUTINE

Do the first seven postures of the sun salutation (see days one through seven) when you get up, followed by the posture below. Walk briskly for 30 to 45 minutes or swim or cycle for 20 minutes. In the evening, unwind in corpse pose (see page 136) for 15 minutes.

SUN SALUTATION—8TH POSTURE

1 After the last pose, exhale and hold your breath. Lower yourself so your toes, chin, chest, and knees touch the floor while keeping your bottom in the air.

2 Relax. Breathe gently in and out. Keep your mind empty.

MEDITATION

Today you will do an advanced chakra meditation that both cleanses and re-energizes your chakras. You will need a small piece of amethyst, diamond, or quartz. These are associated with the crown chakra. Crystals have their own resonance that amplifies the power of meditation.

CHAKRA MEDITATION WITH A CRYSTAL

1 Sit comfortably, holding the crystal in both hands on your lap. Visualize light or "white energy" moving from your base chakra up through your other chakras to your crown chakra.

2 Imagine the light flowing from the crown of your head down through the crystal where it is amplified. Let the light flow back into the base of your spine and up through your chakras to form a continuous flowing wheel of light.

AVOID SLIPS IN MOTIVATION

Motivation can wane after a week of daily aerobic exercise. Keep varying your route, exercise with a friend, and check to see whether your blood pressure has come down.

DAY NINE

DAILY MENU

Breakfast: stuffed tomatoes (see page 226). Slice of wholegrain toast **Morning snack:** a portion of superfood fruit (see day one) **Lunch:** beet and tofu medley (see page 228). Bowl of mixed salad leaves sprinkled with walnuts, pumpkin seeds, chopped garlic, walnut oil, and red wine vinegar. Low-fat yogurt with live cultures with fresh fruit **Afternoon snack:** chocolate petit fours (see page 236) **Dinner:** Thai fish bundles (see page 233). Bok choy. Corn kernels. Almond rice pudding (see page 234)

Drinks: 2½ cups 2% or 1% milk. Freshly squeezed fruit/veg juice. Unlimited green, black, white, or herbal tea, and mineral water. 5 ounces (⅔ cup) red wine or unsweetened red grape juice **Supplements:** see page 200

The bok choy in tonight's dinner is a good source of carotenoids, calcium, magnesium, folic acid, vitamin C, vitamin K, and potassium, making it ideal for hypertension. It can be added raw to salads, lightly steamed, or used in stir-fries. Bok choy with green, rather than white stems, has a higher phytonutrient content.

DAILY EXERCISE ROUTINE

When you get up in the morning do the first eight postures of the sun salutation (see days one through eight) followed by the posture below. Walk briskly for 30 to 45 minutes or swim or cycle for 20 minutes. In the evening, relax in corpse pose (see page 136) for 15 minutes.

SUN SALUTATION—9TH POSTURE

1 Following on from the last pose, let your bottom drop to the floor, lift your chest and stomach, and curl your head back in cobra (see page 135).
2 Hold your breath and stay in the pose for a few seconds, keeping your mind quiet, before starting to breathe gently in and out again.

MEDITATION

Today's meditation is based on a breathing exercise.

BREATH MEDITATION

1 Count how many breaths you take in a minute—it's normally about 12. You're going to try to reduce this to six breaths.

2 Breathe in slowly and deeply through your nose, then out through your mouth. As you inhale, imagine oxygen entering your body through the pores of your skin as well as through your nose so your breathing rate can slow down naturally. At first, try breathing in and out at the same rate—for example, inhale for 5 seconds and exhale for 5 seconds.

3 Now speed up your inhalations and slow your exhalations so you spend around 3 seconds breathing in and 7 seconds breathing out.

4 Focus on emptying your lungs completely, and on keeping air flow continuous. Don't hold your breath between inhaling and exhaling. It takes practice to breathe at the slow rate of just six breaths per minute.

DAY TEN

DAILY MENU

Breakfast: banana-cinnamon oatmeal (see page 141) with coconut shavings

Morning snack: a portion of superfood fruit (see day one)

Lunch: almond and broccoli salad (see page 227). Bowl of mixed salad leaves sprinkled with pumpkin seeds, chopped garlic, walnut oil, and red wine vinegar. Wholewheat roll. Low-fat yogurt with live cultures with fresh fruit

Afternoon snack: beet power juice (see page 236)

Dinner: creamy mushroom cups (see page 229). Red rice. Broccoli. Baked apples (see page 235)

Drinks: 2½ cups 2% or 1% milk. Freshly squeezed fruit/veg juice. Unlimited green, black, white, or herbal tea, and mineral water. 5 ounces (⅔ cup) red wine or unsweetened red grape juice

Supplements: see page 200

Broccoli, in today's lunch, contains antioxidants and substances such as sulforaphane that increase the production of antioxidant detoxification enzymes (glutathiones) throughout the body. These reduce damage to arterial wall linings and help to combat both atherosclerosis and hypertension. Lightly steam broccoli rather than boil to retain maximum nutritional content.

DAILY EXERCISE ROUTINE

When you get up, do the first nine postures of the sun salutation (see days one through nine) followed by the posture below. Walk briskly for 30 to 45 minutes or swim or cycle for 20 minutes. In the evening, lie down in corpse pose (see page 136) for 15 minutes.

SUN SALUTATION—10TH POSTURE

1 Following on from the last posture, breathe out and push up through your feet and hands, lifting your bottom high in the air and straightening your legs.

2 Your body should be in an inverted "V" shape. This is downward dog (see page 131). Tuck your chin into your chest, push your tailbone to the ceiling, and hold your breath. Stay in the position for a few seconds. Keep your mind quiet.

MEDITATION

In today's meditation, I'd like you to focus on raising the temperature of one of your hands. Research using biofeedback machines (see page 65) shows you can use the power of thought to increase blood circulation and temperature in one hand by as much as 5 to 10 degrees. If you can dilate your blood vessels in this way, it can help to lower blood pressure and stop tension headaches.

BODY TEMPERATURE MEDITATION

1 Quietly focus on your dominant hand. Imagine it getting warmer. Direct all your attention to your hand and feel the glow spreading throughout your palm and fingers. Do this for at least 15 minutes.

2 Afterward, place your hands against your cheeks to see if you can feel a temperature difference between them. Alternatively, use a forehead thermometer to measure the skin temperature of each palm.

DAY ELEVEN

DAILY MENU

Breakfast: chopped figs, dates, and apricots mixed with low-fat fromage blanc. Slice of wholegrain, rye, soy, or barley toast
Morning snack: a portion of superfood fruit (see day one)
Lunch: bowl of chopped avocado and low-fat buffalo mozzarella with tomatoes, walnuts, and arugula, dressed with walnut oil and red wine vinegar. Low-fat yogurt with live cultures with fresh fruit
Afternoon snack: a handful of almonds
Dinner: winter vegetable stew with rosemary (see page 232). Pears in red wine (see page 235)
Drinks: 2½ cups 2% or 1% milk. Freshly squeezed fruit/veg juice. Unlimited green, black, white, or herbal tea and mineral water. 5 ounces (⅔ cup) red wine or unsweetened red grape juice
Supplements: see page 200

DAILY EXERCISE ROUTINE

Do the first 10 postures of the sun salutation (see days one through ten) this morning, followed by the posture below. Walk briskly for 30 to 45 minutes or swim or cycle for 20 minutes. In the evening, unwind by lying in the corpse pose (see page 136) for 15 minutes.

SUN SALUTATION—11TH POSTURE

1 Following on straight from the last posture, breathe in and take a big step forward with your left leg so your left foot falls in between your hands.
2 Still breathing in, raise your arms out and up in a wide circle, with your palms coming together above your head, fingers pointing up.
3 Look up at your hands and hold your breath, keeping your mind as empty as possible.

WATCH YOUR PULSE

To help you with today's meditation you can buy a biofeedback device that provides a live readout of your heart rate on your home computer. You can watch your pulse rate fall as you meditate.

MEDITATION

Today I'd like you to focus on slowing your heart rate. Please note that if you're taking a beta-blocker drug you will not be able to influence your heart rate significantly.

HEART-RATE MEDITATION

1 Spend 10 minutes sitting quietly, reading a book or listening to music. Take your pulse rate.
2 Now sit in quiet contemplation but, rather than focusing on a mantra, for example, focus on lowering your heart rate.
3 Imagine your heart beating in your chest. Send it mental signals to beat more slowly.
4 After 10 minutes, take your pulse rate again and see how much it has come down.

DAY TWELVE

DAILY MENU

Breakfast: homemade muesli (see page 141). Banana and walnuts
Morning snack: a portion of superfood fruit (see day one)
Lunch: green minestrone soup (see page 227). Wholewheat roll. Low-fat yogurt with live cultures with fresh fruit
Afternoon snack: raspberry almond smoothie (see page 236)
Dinner: Mediterranean mackerel (see page 233). Wholewheat or hemp pasta. Broccoli. About 1½ ounces dark chocolate

Drinks: 2½ cups 2% or 1% milk. Freshly squeezed fruit/veg juice. Unlimited green, black, white, or herbal tea, and mineral water. 5 ounces (⅔ cup) red wine or unsweetened red grape juice
Supplements: see page 200

The meditations you are doing use principles borrowed from autogenic training and biofeedback (see page 65). Research shows that people with high blood pressure can learn to reduce their blood pressure by 15.3/17.8 mmHg during just three sessions of biofeedback training spread over a two-week period.

DAILY EXERCISE ROUTINE

When you get up, do the first 11 postures of the sun salutation (see days one through eleven) followed by the posture below. Walk briskly for 30 to 45 minutes during the day or swim or cycle for 20 minutes. In the evening, unwind by lying in the corpse pose (see page 136) for 15 minutes.

SUN SALUTATION—12TH POSTURE

1 Following straight on from the 11th posture, breathe out as you bring your right foot forward next to your left foot.
2 Grasp the backs of your ankles or calves (or reach as far down as feels comfortable).
3 Tuck your chin in and bend your elbows to pull your upper body gently in toward your legs.
4 Breathe out and hold your breath for a few seconds while you stay in this pose, keeping your mind as quiet as possible.

MEDITATION

Today I'd like you to focus on lowering your blood pressure.

BLOOD PRESSURE MEDITATION

1 Spend 10 minutes sitting quietly, reading a book, or listening to some music. Then take your blood pressure.
2 Sit in quiet contemplation. Focus on bringing your blood pressure down.
3 Visualize your arteries and veins dilating and imagine your pulse rate and breathing rate gradually becoming slower.
4 After 10 minutes, take your blood pressure again to discover by how much it has come down.

REGULAR BLOOD TESTS

If your cholesterol, triglyceride, and homocysteine levels are in the optimum range, you need to have them checked annually. If they are above optimal, however (or below optimum in the case of good HDL-cholesterol), you might wish to have the nonoptimal values assessed every three to six months.

DAY THIRTEEN

DAILY MENU

Breakfast: oatmeal with Brazil nuts and coconut shavings

Morning snack: a portion of superfood fruit (see day one)

Lunch: cheese, fruit, and nut platter (see page 229). Bowl of mixed salad leaves sprinkled with Brazil nuts, pumpkin seeds, chopped garlic, walnut oil, and red wine vinegar. Low-fat yogurt with live cultures with fresh fruit

Afternoon snack: chocolate florentines (see page 236)

Dinner: lemon pork (see page 232). Spinach. Wholewheat or hemp pasta. Almond rice pudding (see page 234)

Drinks: 2½ cups 2% or 1% milk. Freshly squeezed fruit/veg juice. Unlimited green, black, white, or herbal tea, and mineral water. 5 ounces (⅔ cup) red wine or unsweetened red grape juice

Supplements: see page 200

DAILY EXERCISE ROUTINE

When you get up in the morning do the first 12 postures of the sun salutation (see days one through thirteen) followed by the posture below. Walk briskly for 30 to 45 minutes during the day or swim or cycle for 20 minutes. In the evening, lie down in corpse pose (see page 136) to unwind for 15 minutes.

SUN SALUTATION—13TH POSTURE

1 Following straight on from the last posture, breathe in and straighten up. As you straighten, bring your arms outward and up in a wide circle.
2 Bring your palms together over your head. Point your fingers up, look up at your hands, and lengthen your spine.

PUMPKIN SEEDS

Pumpkin seeds are a nutritious ingredient in today's lunch, and in many other lunches in this program. You can buy pumpkin seeds, but it's also easy to extract them from a pumpkin. Next time you eat pumpkin flesh, take out the seeds and either dry them in a warm oven 3 hours, or toss them with olive oil and roast them 10 minutes at 350°F.

3 Hold your breath and stay in this posture for a few seconds. Keep your mind as empty as possible.

ACUPRESSURE

I introduce you to a new home therapy today: acupressure. Massaging two acupressure points above the nape of your neck can help to bring blood pressure down. These points are on the gall bladder meridian and are called Gb20 (wind pool). To find them, place your thumbs on your earlobes and slide them back toward the base of your skull. They should fall into a small depression on each side of your neck vertebrae, about 1 inch above your hairline. Bend your head forward and back again to find them. Massage these points with firm thumb pressure for a minute. These points are also used to encourage the upward flow of energy through your chakras (see page 61).

DAY FOURTEEN

DAILY MENU

Breakfast: cooked Sunday breakfast (see page 226). Slice of wholegrain, rye, soy, or barley toast
Morning snack: a portion of superfood fruit (see day one)
Lunch: almond trout (see page 228). Bowl of mixed salad leaves sprinkled with cilantro leaves, walnuts, pumpkin seeds, chopped garlic, walnut oil, and red wine vinegar. Low-fat yogurt with live cultures with fresh fruit
Afternoon snack: beet power juice (see page 236)
Dinner: chickpea curry (see page 231). Almond rice pudding (see page 234). About 1½ ounces dark chocolate

Drinks: 2½ cups 2% or 1% milk. Freshly squeezed fruit/veg juice. Unlimited green, black, white, or herbal tea, and mineral water. 5 ounces (⅔ cup) red wine or unsweetened red grape juice
Supplements: see page 200

Once you have learned today's final posture in the sun salutation, you will have a flowing sequence of postures that you can practice every morning. This ancient exercise regime will help you to concentrate and stay calm.

According to yoga adepts, if you can fit in only one yoga exercise per day, it should be the sun salutation.

DAILY EXERCISE ROUTINE

When you get up in the morning do the first 13 postures of the sun salutation (see days one through thirteen) followed by the final posture below. Walk briskly for 30 to 45 minutes during the day, or swim or cycle for 20 minutes. In the evening, unwind by lying down in the corpse pose (see page 136) for 15 minutes.

SUN SALUTATION—14TH POSTURE

1 Following straight on from the 13th posture, breathe out and bring your arms down to your sides in a flowing circle.
2 Bring your palms together in a prayer position in front of your chest. You have now completed a full round of the sun salutation.

CONSULTING AN ACUPUNCTURIST

I suggest that you end the program with a course of traditional Chinese acupuncture. To find an acupuncturist, see page 237. Acupuncture regulates the flow of qi energy in your body and can help to stabilize your blood pressure at a lower level. During a consultation, a practitioner takes your medical history, examines you, and assesses the condition of your tongue, pulse, and tan tien (the area below the navel). Sterile, disposable, slender needles are inserted into the skin over selected acupoints, to a depth of ⅕ inch. This should not be uncomfortable. Usually, between six and 12 needles are used, with points on the hands and feet most commonly selected. Needles can be left in position for as little as a few seconds, while others may be left 30 to 60 minutes. Withdrawal of the needles at the end of the session is usually painless. A course of 12 acupuncture treatments, over a period of six weeks, can significantly lower raised blood pressure, and the effects can last for nine months or more after the final treatment.

CONTINUING THE FULL-STRENGTH PROGRAM

You have just finished two weeks on the full-strength program—well done! I now advise you continue with the eating plan for an additional two weeks. This way you will experience a month of healthy eating and be very familiar with the foods you need to shop for and eat every day. After a month you can then start to vary the foods you eat, and include some new recipes. The following information will help you plan your future on the full-strength program.

YOUR LONG-TERM DIET

The diet you have followed in the full-strength plan is based on heart-friendly superfoods (see pages 80–86). Eating these superfoods on a regular basis means you will significantly reduce your risk of coronary heart disease (see pages 24–25). To continue with this diet:

- Eat at least 2 cups fruit and 2 cups vegetables everyday, along with garlic, almonds, dark chocolate, and red wine or red grape juice.
- Eat fish four times a week (though you can eat less than this if you continue to take garlic and omega-3 fish oil supplements).
- Include as many of the superfoods on pages 80–86 as possible in your daily diet. For example, blueberries, grapes, spinach, and pomegranate.
- Eat mainly vegetarian and fish meals. Research suggests hypertension is linked with a high intake of red and processed meat, whereas whole grains, fruit, nuts, fish, and milk (a rich source of beneficial calcium) have a protective effect on the cardiovascular system. For detailed advice on what to look for when choosing fish and shellfish, see page 181 of the moderate program.
- When you do eat meat, choose poulty or nonfatty cuts of red meat, such as lean pork.

RECIPES

Explore fish-based and vegetarian recipes—you will find delicious recipe suggestions at www.naturalhealthguru.co.uk. You can post your own favorite recipes there for other followers of the program to try. Bear the following points in mind when you're choosing recipes and cooking:

- Look for recipes that include superfoods, such as red wine. Cooking with red wine removes excess alcohol, while retaining useful amounts of antioxidants.
- Include garlic in savory dishes, even if the original recipe doesn't include it.
- Replace salt with freshly ground pepper and freshly chopped herbs.
- Replace cream with yogurt or fromage blanc. For tips on how to use yogurt in cooking, see page 138.

YOUR LONG-TERM SUPPLEMENT REGIME

Continue taking the recommended supplements for the full-strength program (see page 200) long term. Findings from numerous studies back their use at this high level for significant effects on your blood pressure and future health. However, do not increase the doses further without specific, individual advice from a qualified nutritional therapist, naturopath, or doctor. If, up until now, you have taken only the supplements in the recommended list, think about taking one or more of the supplements in the optional list for additional benefits. Full details of each supplement, including updates on latest research findings, are available at www.naturalhealthguru.co.uk.

YOUR EXERCISE ROUTINE

Continue with at least 45 minutes of aerobic exercise per day: brisk walking, cycling, or swimming are ideal. If you don't already belong to a gym, think about joining one—a personal trainer will give you individually tailored advice, help to motivate you, and provide suggestions for improving your muscular fitness as well as your aerobic fitness. Continue to perform the sun salutation every morning when you get up and spend 15 minutes in the corpse pose (see page 136) to wind down at the end of each day. If you enjoy the yoga, consider joining a class or receiving one-to-one tutoring.

YOUR THERAPY PROGRAM

The full-strength program has introduced you to a variety of advanced meditation practices. Continue meditating for at least 20 minutes per day, ideally on two occasions: once in the morning and once in the evening, using whichever of the meditation techniques you find most helpful. You can also attend meditation classes to receive formal instruction from a teacher (read about different types of meditation on page 64).

If you found their interventions helpful, continue to consult the therapists—the naturopath and acupuncturist. Other complementary therapies to consider include biofeedback and autogenic training.

MONITORING YOUR BLOOD PRESSURE

While continuing with the full-strength program, I suggest you monitor your blood pressure on a weekly basis, at the same time of day, unless the doctor has asked you to check it more frequently. Keep a record of your blood pressure measurements in a chart such as the one on page 112. This will give you an instant visual indication of whether your blood pressure is going down (which I would expect during this program), staying the same, or going up.

If your blood pressure is consistently below 130/80 mmHg, well done. The full-strength program has had the desired effect, and, to consolidate the benefits, you should continue it long term. If you're taking prescribed anti-hypertensive medication, your doctor might consider lowering the dose or number of antihypertensive drugs you are taking. This is not something you should do on your own without your doctor's supervision, however. The dose of some anti-hypertensive drugs needs to be reduced slowly to prevent any rebound effects.

If your blood pressure is consistently between 130/80 mmHg and 140/90 mmHg, seek advice from your doctor or naturopath to see if you can bring it down to below 130/80 mmHg. Although a blood pressure of less than 140/90 mmHg is an acceptable target, a level of less than 130/80 mmHg is ideal for long-term health, especially if you also have diabetes or kidney problems. If your blood pressure is consistently above 140/90 mmHg, see your doctor for individual advice.

BREAKFAST RECIPES

BLUEBERRY AND ALMOND MOUSSE

SERVES 4

2½ cups blueberries
10 ounces silken tofu
¾ cup blanched almonds, roughly
    chopped

1 Reserve a few blueberries for serving,
   then place the remainder in a blender
   with the tofu and process until
   smooth.

2 Divide between 4 glass serving bowls.
   Sprinkle the chopped almonds over
   and top with the reserved blueberries.
   Serve.

HERRINGS IN OATS

SERVES 4

4 small herring, dressed, scaled, and
    head and backbone removed
4 tablespoons 2% milk (or almond, rice,
    or soy milk)
4 tablespoons steel-cut oats
2 tablespoons olive oil
Freshly squeezed juice of 1 lime
1 large handful watercress
Freshly ground black pepper

1 Dip the herring in the milk and then roll
   in the oats. Season with black pepper.

2 Heat the oil in a pan. Add the herring
   and fry over low heat about 10
   minutes on each side. Sprinkle each
   fish with a little lime juice and serve
   on a bed of watercress.

WINDWARD ISLANDS TROUT

SERVES 4

4 trout fillets, about 5 ounces each
2 small bananas, peeled and cut in half
    lengthwise
Freshly squeezed juice of 1 orange
Grated peel and freshly squeezed juice
    of 1 unwaxed lemon
1 handful watercress, rinsed and drained
1 handful fresh flat-leaf parsley, roughly
    chopped
Freshly ground black pepper

1 Heat the oven to 350°F.

2 Arrange the trout in a single layer in
   a baking dish. Lay half a banana along
   each fillet and pour the citrus juice
   and peel over. Bake 20 minutes, or
   until the fish is cooked through and
   flakes easily.

3 Season with black pepper and serve
   on a bed of watercress, sprinkled with
   the parsley.

STUFFED TOMATOES

SERVES 4

4 large beefsteak tomatoes
1 shallot, finely chopped
2 garlic cloves, crushed
12 fresh basil leaves, torn
1 handful fresh parsley, chopped
2½ cups sliced mushrooms
1 handful grated mozzarella cheese
  (optional)
Freshly ground black pepper
4 slices wholegrain or rye toast,
  to serve

1 Heat the oven to 350°F.
2 Slice the tops off the tomatoes.
   Scoop out the insides and mix
   with the shallot, garlic, herbs, and
   mushrooms. Season with pepper.
   Stuff the tomatoes with the mixture.
   Top with the cheese (if using),
   replace the tomato tops, and bake
   15 minutes. Serve with toast.

COOKED SUNDAY BREAKFAST

SERVES 4

4 mushrooms, cut in half
4 tomatoes, cut in half
4 small zucchini, cut in half
  lengthwise
1 red bell pepper, seeded and cut into
  8 pieces
1 yellow bell pepper, seeded and cut
  into 8 pieces
4 tablespoons olive oil
4 handfuls spinach leaves, washed
Freshly ground black pepper
4 slices wholegrain toast, to serve

1 Heat the broiler to medium-hot.
2 Put the mushrooms, tomatoes,
   zucchini, and peppers on a baking
   sheet and drizzle with the oil. Put
   under the broiler and broil until
   the vegetables are just tender.
   Meanwhile, cook the spinach leaves
   in a steamer until they wilt.
3 Divide the broiled vegetables and
   spinach between 4 warm serving
   plates. Season with black pepper
   and serve with the toast.

LUNCH RECIPES

GREEN MINESTRONE

SERVES 4

1 tablespoon olive oil
1 onion, chopped
1 leek, chopped
4 garlic cloves, crushed
1 quart vegetable stock (see page 153)
  or water
3½ ounces green lasagne sheets,
  broken into bite-size pieces
⅔ cup broccoli florets
¾ cup shelled peas, fresh or frozen
2 cups shredded leafy greens, such as
  spinach, kale, savoy cabbage, or
  bok choy
1 zucchini, finely chopped
1 handful fresh basil leaves, shredded
Freshly ground black pepper

1　Heat the oil in a large skillet. Add the
   onion, leek, and garlic and cook over
   medium heat until soft. Pour in the
   vegetable stock and bring to a boil.
   Add the green pasta pieces and cook
   5 minutes.

2　Add the broccoli, peas, shredded
   greens, and zucchini and simmer
   gently 3 minutes longer. Stir in
   the basil leaves, season with black
   pepper, and serve.

ALMOND AND BROCCOLI SALAD

SERVES 4

3 cups broccoli florets
4 tablespoons walnut or extra virgin
  olive oil
3 tablespoons lemon juice
1 garlic clove, crushed
2 sprigs oregano or thyme, leaves
  chopped
Freshly ground black pepper
4 large scallions, roughly chopped
Scant 1 cup slivered almonds, lightly
  toasted

1　Plunge the broccoli into a pan of
   boiling water. Return to the boil
   and boil 1 minute; drain and then
   plunge into cold water.

2　Put the oil, lemon juice, garlic,
   and oregano in a small bowl and
   mix well; season with black pepper.

3　Toss the broccoli, scallions, and
   almonds in a large serving bowl.
   Pour the oil and lemon mixture
   over and serve.

BEET AND TOFU MEDLEY

SERVES 4

2 cups cubed firm tofu
1½ cups peeled and cubed cooked
  baby beets
1 small red onion, thinly sliced
1 ripe avocado, peeled, pitted, and
  flesh roughly chopped
Freshly squeezed juice of 1 lime
2 tablespoons walnut or extra virgin
  olive oil
2 teaspoons wholegrain mustard
3½ cups mixed baby salad leaves
Freshly ground black pepper

1 Mix the tofu, beet, onion, and
   avocado in a bowl; set aside.

2 Put the lime juice, oil, and mustard
   in a screw-top jar and shake until
   thoroughly mixed. Pour over the
   tofu and beet mixture and toss well.

3 Put the salad leaves in a serving
   bowl and top with the tofu and
   beet mixture. Season with pepper
   and serve.

ALMOND TROUT

SERVES 4

4 trout fillets, about 7 ounces each
4 tablespoons 2% milk (or almond, rice,
  or soymilk)
4 tablespoons ground blanched almonds
2 tablespoons olive oil
4 tomatoes, cut in half
4 tablespoons slivered almonds, lightly
  toasted
Freshly ground black pepper

1 Dip the trout in the milk and roll in
   the ground almonds.

2 Heat the oil in a large skillet. Add
   the tomatoes and trout and cook
   over low heat about 4 minutes on
   each side, until the fish is cooked
   through.

3 Arrange the trout and tomatoes on
   4 warm serving plates. Season with
   pepper, sprinkle with the almonds,
   and serve.

DINNER RECIPES

CHEESE, FRUIT AND NUT PLATTER

SERVES 4

9 ounces mixed salad leaves

2 handfuls watercress

2 oranges, peeled, pith removed, and thinly sliced

1 small pineapple, peeled, cored, and thinly sliced

1 kiwi, peeled and thinly sliced

1¼ cups cottage cheese

1 cup walnuts

Scant 1 cup mixed seeds, such as flax seed, sunflower, pumpkin, and sesame

1　Put the salad leaves and watercress on a large serving dish and arrange the fruit on top.

2　Mix the cottage cheese, walnuts, and seeds in a bowl. Pile this mixture on top of the fruit and serve.

CREAMY MUSHROOM CUPS

SERVES 4

1 shallot, finely chopped

1 handful fresh parsley, roughly chopped

5 ounces silken tofu

Grated peel and freshly squeezed juice of 1 unwaxed lemon

Freshly ground black pepper

12 small mushrooms, stems removed

1 teaspoon paprika

1 handful mixed salad leaves, to serve

1　Put the shallot, parsley, and tofu in a bowl and mash together to form a paste. Stir in the lemon juice and peel and season with black pepper.

2　Put the mushrooms, hollow-side up, on a serving platter. Pile the tofu mixture into the mushrooms, sprinkle each one with a little paprika, and serve with the salad leaves.

MEDITERRANEAN HERB OIL

2½ cups extra virgin olive oil
12 black peppercorns
12 green peppercorns
12 fennel seeds
12 coriander seeds
2 sprigs rosemary
2 sprigs thyme
2 sprigs tarragon
2 sprigs oregano
2 bay leaves
2 fresh red chilies, scored lengthwise

1 Put all the ingredients in a clear wine
   bottle. Cork to form a tight seal and
   shake well.

2 Put in a warm place, such as a sunny
   windowsill, and leave for at least
   2 weeks, shaking and turning the
   bottle every day. Use as required.

ORIENTAL TOFU STIR-FRY

SERVES 4

1 tablespoon olive oil
4 garlic cloves, crushed
2-inch piece gingerroot, peeled and
   grated
14 ounces firm tofu, cut into ¾-inch
   cubes
2 cups broccoli florets
1½ cups snow peas or sugar-snap peas
3 cups coarsely shredded bok choy
1½ cups bean sprouts
1 quart vegetable stock (see page 153)
Freshly ground black pepper
2 tablespoons slivered almonds
1 handful fresh cilantro leaves, roughly
   chopped

1 Swirl the olive oil in a hot skillet
   or wok. Add the garlic and ginger
   and stir-fry over high heat 1 minute.
   Toss in the tofu, broccoli, peas, bok
   choy, and bean sprouts and stir-fry
   3 minutes longer.

2 Pour in the stock, bring to a boil,
   and simmer 2 minutes. Season with
   pepper, sprinkle with the slivered
   almonds and cilantro leaves, and
   serve.

ALMOND RICE

SERVES 4

1½ teaspoons olive oil

1 onion, chopped

2 garlic cloves

1 cup long-grain brown or red rice

1 handful raisins

2½ cups vegetable stock (see page 153)

1 handful slivered almonds

1 handful fresh flat-leaf parsley, roughly
  chopped

1 Heat the oil in a pan. Add the onion
  and garlic and fry over medium heat
  until soft. Add the rice and stir-fry
  1 minute. Meanwhile, heat the stock
  in a separate pan.

2 Stir the raisins into the rice, pour
  the hot stock over and bring to a boil.
  Lower the heat, cover, and simmer
  gently, stirring occasionally, about
  30 minutes, or until the rice is tender
  and all the liquid is absorbed. If the
  rice needs longer cooking, add a little
  more stock or water and continue
  until the rice is tender.

3 Remove the pan from the heat. Fold
  in the almonds and parsley and serve
  hot or cold.

CHICKPEA CURRY

SERVES 4

1 tablespoon extra virgin olive oil

1 onion, chopped

4 garlic cloves, crushed

2-inch piece gingerroot, peeled and
  grated

2 tablespoons coriander seeds, crushed
  or ground

1 tablespoon cumin seeds, ground

1 to 2 fresh red chilies, seeded and finely
  chopped

1 large tomato, skinned, seeded, and
  chopped

1½ cups sliced mushrooms

1 can (15-oz.) chickpeas, drained

¾ cup coconut milk

Freshly squeezed juice of 1 lime

1 to 2 handfuls fresh cilantro leaves,
  roughly chopped

1 handful slivered almonds, lightly
  toasted

Freshly ground black pepper

1 Heat the oil in a pan. Add the onion
  and cook over medium heat about
  3 minutes until soft. Add the garlic,
  ginger, coriander, cumin seeds, and
  chilies and stir-fry another 3 minutes.
  Add the tomato and mushrooms and
  cook 5 minutes longer.

2 Add the chickpeas, coconut milk,
  lime juice, and 1 handful cilantro
  and simmer 10 minutes. Season with
  pepper and sprinkle with the almonds
  and another handful cilantro.

WINTER VEGETABLE STEW WITH ROSEMARY
SERVES 4

2 butternut squash, or half a large
    pumpkin, peeled, seeded, and chopped
1 quart vegetable stock (see page 153)
    or water
1 onion, chopped
1 bay leaf
1 handful rosemary sprigs
1 tablespoon extra virgin olive oil
2 leeks, chopped
4 garlic cloves, crushed
1 parsnip, chopped
2 sweet potatoes, chopped
1½ cups canned lima beans, drained
Freshly ground black pepper

1 Put half the squash in a pan with
   the stock, onion, bay leaf, and most
   of the rosemary (set aside a few
   sprigs to serve). Bring to a boil,
   lower the heat, and leave to simmer
   30 minutes. Remove the bay leaf,
   allow to cool a little, then purée in
   a blender; set aside.

2 Heat the oil in a clean pan. Add the
   leeks and garlic and stir-fry until soft.
   Add the remaining squash, parsnip,
   and sweet potatoes and stir-fry
   5 minutes longer.

3 Stir in the lima beans and puréed
   squash and leave to simmer 30
   minutes. Season with pepper and
   serve with rosemary sprigs.

LEMON PORK
SERVES 4

1 shallot, chopped
4 garlic cloves
1 tablespoon olive oil
4 lean pork tenderloins, about
    6 ounces each, cut into cubes
1 tablespoon cumin seeds, crushed
1 tablespoon coriander seeds, crushed
1¼ cups light red wine
1 lemon, thinly sliced
Freshly ground black pepper

1 Cook the shallot and garlic in the oil.
   Add the pork and cumin and coriander
   seeds and stir gently to brown the meat.

2 Add half the wine and simmer gently
   25 minutes. Stir in the lemon and
   remaining wine. Season with pepper
   and serve.

MACKEREL AND CUCUMBER IN WINE
SERVES 4

½ small cucumber, sliced
4 mackerel fillets, about 5 ounces each
1 handful fresh dill or flat-leaf parsley,
    roughly chopped
Scant ½ cup dry white wine
Freshly ground black pepper

1 Heat the oven to 350°F.

2 Line a baking dish with the cucumber.
   Add the other ingredients, cover, and
   bake 30 minutes. Serve.

MEDITERRANEAN MACKEREL

SERVES 4

1½ teaspoons olive oil
1 onion, chopped
2 garlic cloves, chopped
2 cups skinned, seeded, and chopped
   tomatoes
Freshly squeezed juice and grated peel
   of 1 large unwaxed lemon
1 bay leaf
4 mackerel fillets, about 5 ounces each
Freshly ground black pepper
1 handful fresh flat-leaf parsley, roughly
   chopped

1 Preheat the broiler to hot.

2 Heat the oil in a pan. Add the onion
   and garlic and cook over medium
   heat 5 minutes until soft. Add the
   tomatoes, lemon juice and peel, and
   bay leaf, cover, and leave to simmer
   gently about 15 minutes.

3 Meanwhile, put the mackerel fillets
   in a single layer on a baking sheet,
   season with pepper, and broil about
   10 minutes, turning halfway through
   the cooking time.

4 Put the broiled mackerel on 4 warm
   serving plates. Top each one with
   tomato sauce, sprinkle with parsley,
   and serve.

THAI FISH BUNDLES

SERVES 4

1 lemongrass stalk, peeled and finely
   chopped
4 garlic cloves, crushed
2 shallots, chopped
Freshly squeezed juice and grated peel
   of 1 unwaxed lime
1½ tablespoon extra virgin or olive oil
1 fresh green chili, seeded and chopped
1 fresh red chili, seeded and chopped
1 handful fresh cilantro leaves, roughly
   chopped
4 sea bass fillets, about 7 ounces each

1 Heat the oven to 350°F.

2 Put the lemongrass, garlic, shallots,
   lime juice and peel, oil, chilies, and
   cilantro leaves in a blender and
   process to form a paste.

3 Lay each fish fillet in the middle of
   a piece of foil, large enough to wrap
   around it to form a sealed bundle.
   Spread one-quarter of the spicy
   mixture over the top of each piece
   of fish and fold up the foil to form
   4 well-sealed bundles. Put the
   bundles on a baking sheet and bake
   15 minutes.

DESSERT RECIPES

ALMOND RICE PUDDING
SERVES 4

1 cup long-grain brown rice
1 quart almond milk
1 cinnamon stick
1 handful slivered almonds
1 handful dried dates, chopped
(optional)

1 Put the rice, almond milk, and cinnamon stick in a pan and bring to a boil. Lower the heat, cover, and leave to simmer gently 40 minutes, stirring occasionally, until the rice is tender and all the liquid is absorbed.

2 Serve hot or cold, sprinkled with the slivered almonds and chopped dates, if using.

ALMOND-CHOCOLATE CUPS
SERVES 4

3½ ounces dark chocolate, plus extra grated chocolate to serve
9 ounces silken tofu
1 handful ground blanched almonds
1 handful slivered almonds

1 Melt the chocolate. Using a pastry brush, paint the chocolate over the sides and bases of 4 paper muffin liners, so each has a thick chocolate lining. Put in the refrigerator. When hard, peel off the paper case.

2 Process the tofu and ground almonds in a blender. Fill the chocolate cups with this mixture, then chill. Serve sprinkled with the slivered almonds and grated chocolate.

PEARS IN RED WINE

SERVES 4

4 firm pears
1 cinnamon stick
1¼ cups fruity red wine, such as
    Beaujolais
1 tablespoon honey (optional)
Low-fat fromage blanc, to serve

1 Heat the oven to 350°F.

2 Halve each pear lengthwise and
   scoop out the core. Thinly pare away
   the skin. Put the pears in a baking
   dish with the cinnamon stick. Pour
   the red wine over and carefully stir
   in the honey, if using.

3 Cover the dish with foil and bake
   20 minutes. Remove from the oven,
   turn the pears over, re-cover with foil,
   then return to the oven and cook
   20 minutes longer until the pears are
   tender. Serve hot or chilled with the
   fromage blanc.

BAKED APPLES

SERVES 4

4 large apples, such as Jonathan
1 handful slivered almonds
1 handful walnuts, roughly chopped
1 small handful raisins
Freshly squeezed juice and peel of
    1 unwaxed lemon
1¼ cups white wine
Low-fat fromage blanc, to serve

1 Heat the oven to 350°F.

2 Cut the cores out of the apples,
   leaving them whole. With a sharp
   knife, cut just through the skin around
   the middle of each fruit. Stand the
   apples upright in a baking dish.

3 Mix together the almonds, walnuts,
   raisins, and lemon juice and peel
   in a small bowl. Stuff a little of this
   mixture into the hollow in the middle
   of each apple. Pour a little wine over
   each apple.

4 Bake 30 minutes, basting occasionally
   with the juices, until the apples are
   tender. Serve hot with fromage blanc.

BITES, SNACKS AND DRINKS

TOASTED ALMONDS WITH SEEDS
SERVES 4

1 handful blanched almonds
1 handful pumpkin seeds
1 handful sunflower seeds
1 handful flax seeds
1 handful raisins (optional)

1 Toast the almonds and the seeds in a dry pan for a few seconds, stirring until they turn golden brown.

2 Let the nuts and seeds cool in a shallow dish. Mix in the raisins, if using, and serve.

RASPBERRY ALMOND SMOOTHIE
SERVES 4

2½ cups almond milk
4 handfuls fresh raspberries
2 handfuls crushed ice
Fresh mint leaves, to serve

1 Put all the ingredients, except the mint, in a blender and process until smooth.

2 Pour into 4 tall serving glasses. Top with the mint leaves and serve immediately.

CHOCOLATE PETIT FOURS
SERVES 4

4 ounces seedless black grapes
⅔ cup Brazil nuts
3 ounces dark chocolate, melted

1 Dip each grape and nut into the chocolate. Chill until set.

CHOCOLATE FLORENTINES
SERVES 4

7 ounces dark chocolate, melted
1 handful slivered almonds
1 handful dried cranberries
Grated peel of 1 unwaxed lemon

1 Drop small spoonfuls of chocolate onto waxed paper. Top each chocolate circle with almonds, cranberries, and lemon peel. Chill until set.

BEET POWER JUICE
SERVES 4

3 cups roughly chopped raw beets
4 carrots, peeled and roughly chopped
4 oranges, peeled and roughly chopped
1 handful crushed ice

1 Juice the beet, carrots, and oranges; mix. Serve with ice.

RESOURCES

Visit **www.naturalhealthguru.co.uk** for more information, medical references and to post questions or comments about the Natural Health Guru programs.

Blood pressure and stroke
American Heart Association
www.heart.org/heartorg

Canadian Hypertension Society
www.hypertension.ca

National Institutes of Health
www.nih.gov

American Stroke Association
www.strokeassociation.org

Salt
Consensus Action on Salt
and Health (CASH)
www.actionsalt.org.uk

Aromatherapy
USA: National Association
of Holistic Aromatherapy
www.naha.org

Acupuncture
American Association
of Oriental Medicine
www.aaom.org

American Academy of Medical
Acupuncture
www.medicalacupuncture.org

Chinese Medicine and
Acupuncture Association
of Canada
www.cmaac.ca

Herbal medicine
American Herbal Pharmacopoeia
www.herbal-ahp.org

International Register
of Consultant Herbalists
and Homeopaths
www.irch.org

Ontario Herbalists Association
www.herbalists.on.ca

Homeopathy
American Institute
of Homeopathy
www.homeopathyusa.org

Canadian National United
Professional Association
of Trained Homeopaths
www.nupath.org

North American Society
of Homeopaths
www.homeopathy.org

Naturopathy
American Association of
Naturopathic Physicians
www.naturopathic.org

American Naturopathic
Medical Association
www.anma.com

Canadian College
of Naturopathic Medicine
www.ccnm.edu

Reflexology
Reflexology Association
of America
www.reflexology-usa.org

Reflexology Association
of Canada
www.reflexology.org.ca

Yoga
American Yoga Association
www.americanyogaassociation.org

Canadian Yoga Alliance
www.canadianyogicalliance.com

Healthy eating
National Heart, Lung,
and Blood Institute
Your guide to lowering blood
pressure with DASH (enter
"DASH" in the search field)
www.nhlbi.nih.gov

USDA Food Pyramid
www.mypyramid.gov

American Dietetic Association
www.eatright.org

United States Department
of Agriculture's Food and
Nutrition Information Center
www.nutrition.gov

Smoking and alcohol
The Foundation for
a Smokefree America
www.anti-smoking.org

National Institute on
Alcohol Abuse and Alcoholism
www.niaaa.nih.gov

INDEX